Lean & Green

Cookbook

250+ Delicious Recipes to stay **HEALTHY** and **FIT**!

Easy Green Meals Recipes for **Rapid Weight loss**!

<u>**Save your time in kitchen**</u> with Green cooking!

By

Michelle Laurie Johnson

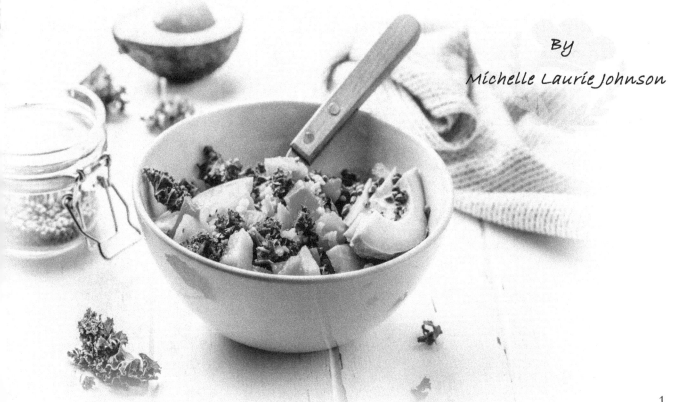

Table of Content

BOOK 1: LEAN & GREEN DAILY RECIPES 4

INTRODUCTION 5

BREAKFAST AND SNACK RECIPES 7

SPECIAL LUNCH RECIPES 25

DINNER RECIPES...36

BOOK 2: DELICIOUS RECIPES AND 21-DAY MEAL PLAN.....................41

SOUP AND STEW RECIPES...42

VEGETABLES...54

SALAD RECIPES 59

SEAFOOD...69

LEAN AND GREEN RECIPES..73

DELICIOUS RECIPES 79

DESSERT...87

NUTRIENT PROTEIN SALAD RECIPES 99

21 DAY MEAL PLAN 103

CONCLUSION..104

BOOK 1: LEAN & GREEN DAILY RECIPES

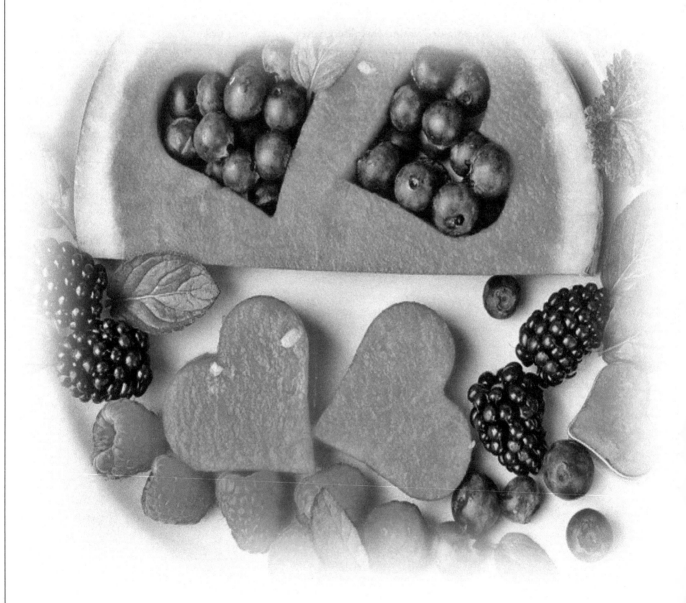

Introduction

"We are what we Eat."

For many years we have listened to this sentence, passed on from our grandparents to us.

It is simply the truth: **our body works because we give it the right fuel by eating foods.** Scientists said that to prevent pathologies such as heart disease, diabetes and cancer, we must eat the right amount of nutrients every day. **I agree with them and this is the reason why I created this book!**

We are obsessed with the diet of the moment, and the media bombards us with the right diet to follow. Many people change their diet during the course of their lives due to their health needs: due to renal disease, diabetes, hypertension of food intolerances.

	Federal Government Recommendation	
Calories	**Men** 19-25: 2,800 26-45: 2,600 46-65: 2,400 65+: 2,200	**Women** 19-25: 2,200 26-50: 2,000 51+: 1,800
Total fat (% of Calorie Intake)	20%-35%	
Total Carbohydrates (% of Calorie Intake)	45%-65%	
Sugars	N/A	
Fiber	**Men** 19-30: 34 g. 31-50: 31 g. 51+: 28 g.	**Women** 19-30: 28 g. 31-50: 25 g. 51+: 22 g
Protein	10%-35%	
Sodium	Under 2,300 mg.	
Potassium	At least 4,700 mg.	
Calcium	**Men** 1,000 mg.	**Women** 19-50: 1,000 mg. 51+: 1,200 mg

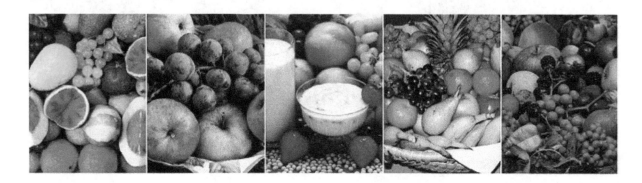

Regardless of the diet you follow currently, the recipes you will find in this book may be for you, because they are all healthy and lean!

Lean & Green recipes are the building blocks for creating the right habits and meals for any diet!

If your goal is to stay healthy, prevent heart disease, prevent diabetes and cancer these recipes could help you assume the amount of the right nutrients.

Every recipe in this book contains the right amount of nutrients according to the **Federal Government Recommendation** and each of them **can be a part of your diet plan you are following**.

What could be better than a cookbook with light recipes when the imagination is scarce in the kitchen?

That way, you can cook and stay fit, without sacrificing taste!

I wish you a good read and... good cooking!

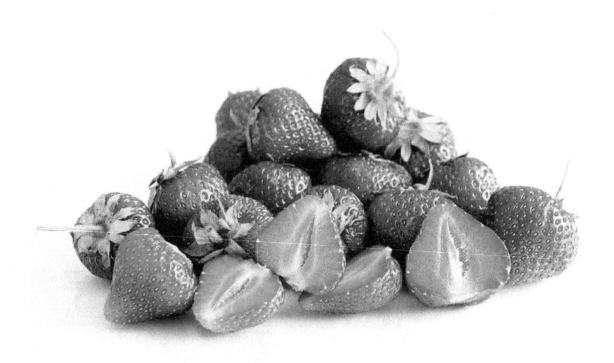

Breakfast and Snack Recipes

TASTY BREAKFAST DONUTS

Preparation Time: 5 minutes

Cooking Time: 5 minutes

Servings: 4

Ingredients:

- 43 grams' cream cheese
- 2 eggs
- 2 tablespoons almond flour
- 2 tablespoons erythritol
- 1 ½ tablespoons coconut flour
- ½ teaspoon baking powder
- ½ teaspoon vanilla extract
- 5 drops Stevia (liquid form)
- 2 strips bacon, fried until crispy

Directions:
1. Rub coconut oil over donut maker and turn on.
2. Pulse all ingredients except bacon in a blender or food processor until smooth (should take around 1 minute).
3. Pour batter into donut maker, leaving 1/10 in each round for rising.
4. Leave for 3 minutes before flipping each donut. Leave for another 2 minutes or until fork comes out clean when piercing them. Take donuts out and let them cool.
5. Repeat steps 1-5 until all batter is used.
6. Crumble bacon into bits and use to top donuts.

CHEESY SPICY BACON BOWLS

Preparation Time: 10 minutes
Cooking Time: 22 minutes
Servings: 12
Ingredients:

- 6 strips Bacon, pan fried until cooked but still malleable
- 4 eggs
- 60 grams' cheddar cheese
- 40 grams' cream cheese, grated
- 2 Jalapenos, sliced and seeds removed
- 2 tablespoons coconut oil
- ¼ teaspoon onion powder
- ¼ teaspoon garlic powder
- Dash of salt and pepper

Directions:
1. Preheat oven to 375°F.
2. In a bowl, beat together eggs, cream cheese, jalapenos (minus 6 slices), coconut oil, onion powder, garlic powder, and salt and pepper. Using leftover bacon grease on a muffin tray, rubbing it into each insert. Place bacon wrapped inside the parameters of each insert.
3. Pour beaten mixture halfway up each bacon bowl.
4. Garnish each bacon bowl with cheese and leftover jalapeno slices (placing one on top of each).
5. Leave in the oven for about 22 minutes, or until egg is thoroughly cooked and cheese is bubbly.
6. Remove from oven and let cool until edible. Enjoy!

GOAT CHEESE ZUCCHINI KALE QUICHE

Preparation Time: 35 minutes
Cooking Time: 1 hour 10 minutes
Servings: 4
Ingredients:

- 4 large eggs
- 8 ounces' fresh zucchini, sliced
- 10 ounces' kale
- 3 garlic cloves (minced)
- 1 cup soymilk
- 1 ounce's goat cheese
- 1cup grated parmesan
- 1cup shredded cheddar cheese
- 2 teaspoons olive oil
- Salt and pepper, to taste

Directions:

1. Preheat oven to 350°F.
2. Heat 1 tsp of olive oil in a saucepan over medium-high heat. Sauté garlic for 1 minute until flavored.
3. Add the zucchini and cook for another 5-7 minutes until soft.
4. Beat the eggs and then add a little milk and Parmesan cheese.
5. Meanwhile, heat the remaining olive oil in another saucepan and add the cabbage. Cover and cook for 5 minutes until dry. Slightly grease a baking dish with cooking spray and spread the kale leaves across the bottom. Add the zucchini and top with goat cheese.
6. Pour the egg, milk and parmesan mixture evenly over the other ingredients. Top with cheddar cheese.
7. Bake for 50–60 minutes until golden brown. Check the center of the quiche, it should have a solid consistency.
8. Let chill for a few minutes before serving.

CREAM CHEESE EGG BREAKFAST

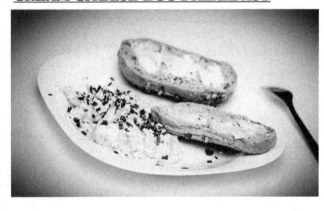

Servings: 4   **Preparation Time:** 5 minutes

Ingredients: **Cooking Time:** 5 minutes

- 2 eggs, beaten
- 1 tablespoon butter
- 2 tablespoons soft cream cheese with chives

Directions:
1. Melt the butter in a small skillet.
2. Add the eggs and cream cheese.
3. Stir and cook to desired doneness.

AVOCADO RED PEPPERS ROASTED SCRAMBLED EGGS

Preparation Time: 10 minutes
Cooking Time: 12 minutes
Servings: 3
Ingredients:
- 1/2 tablespoon butter
- Eggs, 2
- 1/2 roasted red pepper, about 1 1/2 ounces
- 1/2 small avocado, coarsely chopped, about 2 1/4 ounces
- Salt, to taste

Directions:
1. In a nonstick skillet, heat the butter over medium heat. Break the eggs into the pan and break the yolks with a spoon. Sprinkle with a little salt.
2. Stir and continue stirring until the eggs start to come out. Quickly add the bell peppers and avocado.
3. Cook and stir until the eggs suit your taste. Adjust the seasoning, if necessary. Serve!

MUSHROOM QUICKIE SCRAMBLE

Preparation Time: 10 minutes
Cooking Time: 10 minutes
Servings: 4
Ingredients:
- 3 small sized eggs, whisked
- 4 pcs. Bella mushrooms
- ½ cup of spinach
- ¼ cup of red bell peppers
- 2 deli ham slices
- 1 tablespoon of ghee or coconut oil
- Salt and pepper to taste

Directions:
1. Chop the ham and veggies.

2. Put half a tbsp of butter in a frying pan and heat until melted.
3. Sauté the ham and vegetables in a frying pan then set aside.
4. Get a new frying pan and heat the remaining butter.
5. Add the whisked eggs into the second pan while stirring continuously to avoid overcooking.
6. When the eggs are done, sprinkle with salt and pepper to taste.
7. Add the ham and veggies to the pan with the eggs. Mix well.
8. Remove from burner and transfer to a plate. Serve and enjoy.

COCONUT COFFEE AND GHEE

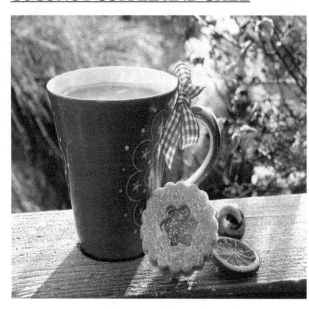

Preparation Time: 10 minutes
Cooking Time: 10 minutes
Servings: 5
Ingredients:
- ½ Tbsp. of coconut oil
- ½ Tbsp. of ghee
- 1 to 2 cups of preferred coffee (or rooibos or black tea)
- 1 Tbsp. of coconut or almond milk

Directions:
1. Place the almond (or coconut) milk, coconut oil, ghee and coffee in a blender (or milk frothier).
2. mix for around 10 seconds or until the coffee turns creamy and foamy.
3. Pour contents into a coffee cup.
4. Serve immediately and enjoy.

YUMMY VEGGIE WAFFLES

Preparation Time: 10 minutes
Cooking Time: 9 minutes
Servings: 3
Ingredients:
- 3 cups raw cauliflower, grated
- 1 cup cheddar cheese
- 1 cup mozzarella cheese
- ½ cup parmesan
- 1/3 cup chives, finely sliced
- 6 eggs
- 1 teaspoon garlic powder
- 1 teaspoon onion powder
- ½ teaspoon chili flakes
- Dash of salt and pepper

Directions:
1. Turn waffle maker on. In a bowl mix all the listed ingredients very well until incorporated. Once waffle maker is hot, distribute waffle mixture into the insert.
2. Let cook for about 9 minutes, flipping at 6 minutes.
3. Remove from waffle maker and set aside.
4. Repeat the previous steps with the rest of the batter until gone (should come out to 4 waffles).
5. Serve and enjoy!

OMEGA 3 BREAKFAST SHAKE

Preparation Time: 5 minutes
Cooking Time: 5 minutes
Servings: 2
Ingredients:

- 1 cup vanilla almond milk (unsweetened)
- 2 tablespoons blueberries
- 1 ½ tablespoons flaxseed meal
- 1 tablespoon MCT Oil
- ¾ tablespoon banana extract
- ½ tablespoon chia seeds
- 5 drops Stevia (liquid form)
- 1/8 tablespoon Xanthan gum

Directions:

1. In a blender, pulse vanilla almond milk, banana extract, Stevia, and 3 ice cubes.
2. When smooth, add blueberries and pulse.
3. Once blueberries are thoroughly incorporated, add flaxseed meal and chia seeds.
4. Let sit for 5 minutes. After 5 minutes, pulse again until all ingredients are nicely distributed. Serve and enjoy

LIME BACON THYME MUFFINS

Preparation Time: 10 minutes
Cooking Time: 20 minutes
Servings: 3
Ingredients:

- 3 cups of almond flour
- 4 medium-sized eggs
- 1 cup of bacon bits
- 2 tsp. of lemon thyme
- ½ cup of melted ghee
- 1 tsp. of baking soda
- ½ tsp. of salt, to taste

Directions:

1. Pre-heat oven to 350° F.
2. Put ghee in mixing bowl and melt. Add baking soda and almond flour. Put the eggs in. Add the lemon thyme (if preferred, other herbs or spices may be used). Drizzle with salt. Mix all ingredients well. Sprinkle with bacon bits.
3. Line the muffin pan with liners.
4. Spoon mixture into the pan, filling the pan to about ¾ full. Bake for about 20 minutes. Test by inserting a toothpick into a muffin.
5. If it comes out clean, then the muffins are done. Serve immediately.

GLUTEN -FREE PANCAKES

Preparation Time: 5 minutes
Cooking Time: 2 minutes
Servings: 2
Ingredients:

- 6 eggs
- 1 cup low-fat cream cheese
- 1 1/2 teaspoons baking powder
- 1 scoop protein powder
- 1/4; cup almond meal
- ¼ teaspoon salt
- 2 tablespoons coconut oil
- Fresh currant
- 1 peach
- Powder sugar (optional)

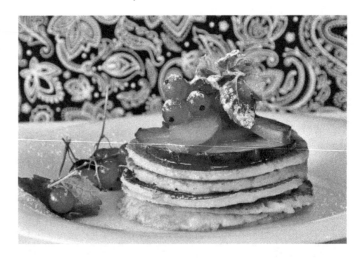

Directions:

1. Take a food processor and combine baking powder, almond flour and salt. Blend for 1 minutes, then add the eggs one after another and then the cream cheese. Blend until smooth.
2. Lightly grease a skillet with coconut oil and place over medium-high heat.
3. Pour the batter into the pan. Turn the pan gently to create round pancakes.
4. Cook for about 2 minutes on each side.
5. Garnish with sliced peach, currant and powder sugar and serve pancakes!

MUSHROOM AND SPINACH OMELET

Preparation Time: 20 minutes
Cooking Time: 20 minutes
Servings: 3
Ingredients:

- 2 tablespoons butter, divided
- 6-8 fresh mushrooms, sliced, 5 ounces
- Chives, chopped, optional
- Salt and pepper, to taste
- 1 handful baby spinach, about 1/2 ounce
- Pinch garlic powder
- 4 eggs, beaten
- 1-ounce shredded Swiss cheese

Directions:

1. In a very large saucepan, sauté the mushrooms in 1 tablespoon of butter until soft. season with salt, pepper and garlic.
2. Remove the mushrooms from the pan and keep warm. Heat the remaining tablespoon of butter in the same skillet over medium heat.
3. Beat the eggs with a little salt and pepper and add to the hot butter. Turn the pan over to coat the entire bottom of the pan with egg. Once the egg is almost out, place the cheese over the middle of the tortilla.
4. Fill the cheese with spinach leaves and hot mushrooms. Let cook for about a minute for the spinach to start to wilt. Fold the empty side of the tortilla carefully over the filling and slide it onto a plate and sprinkle with chives, if desired.
5. Alternatively, you can make two tortillas using half the mushroom, spinach, and cheese filling in each.

PROTEIN OATCAKES

Preparation Time: 10 minutes
Cooking Time: 5 minutes
Servings: 1
Ingredients:

- 70g oatmeal
- 15g protein
- 1 egg white
- ½ cup water
- ½ teaspoon cinnamon
- 60g curd
- 1 teaspoon cacao powder
- 15g sugar

Directions:

1. Mix the oatmeal, protein, egg white, and water in a bowl.
2. Preheat a saucepan to medium heat.
3. Place the mixture into the saucepan.
4. While waiting, prepare the topping by mixing the curd, cinnamon, and sugar in a second bowl.
5. Remove the oatcake from the saucepan when it becomes golden-brown.
6. Add the topping and cocoa powder.
7. Serve on a plate.

ORANGE RICOTTA PANCAKES

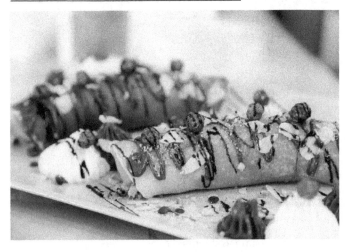

Preparation Time: 10 minutes
Cooking Time: 5 minutes
Servings: 1
Ingredients:

- ¾ cup all-purpose flour
- ½ tablespoon baking powder
- 2 teaspoons sugar
- ½ teaspoon salt
- 3 separated eggs
- 1 cup fresh ricotta
- ¾ cup whole milk
- ½ teaspoon pure vanilla extract
- 1 large ripe orange

Directions:
1. Mix the flour, baking powder, sugar in a large bowl. Add a pinch of salt.
2. In a separate bowl, whisk egg yolk, ricotta, milk, orange zest, and orange juice.
3. Add some vanilla extract for additional flavor. Followed by the dry ingredients to the ricotta mixture and mix adequately. Stir the egg white in a different bowl, and then gently fold it in the ricotta mixture.
4. Preheat saucepan to medium heat and brush with some butter until evenly spread.
5. Use a measuring cup to drop the batter onto the saucepan, ensure the pan is not crowded.
6. Allow cooking for 2 minutes. Flip the food when you notice the edges begin to set, and bubbles form in the center. Cook the meat for another 1 to 2 minutes. Serve with any toppings of your choice.

ASIAN SCRAMBLED EGG

Preparation Time: 10 minutes
Cooking Time: 10 minutes
Servings: 1
Ingredients:

- 1 large egg
- 1/2 teaspoons light soy sauce
- 1/8 teaspoon white pepper
- 1 tablespoon vegetable oil

Directions:
1. Beat the eggs in a bowl. Add soy sauce, one-teaspoon vegetable oil, and pepper.
2. Heat olive oil in a saucepan on medium. Then add the mixture of the beaten egg.
3. The edges will begin to cook. Lessen the heat to medium and carefully scramble the eggs.
4. Turn off heat and transfer into a bowl. Serve hot and enjoy!

ARTICHOKE FRITTATAS

Preparation Time: 10 minutes
Cooking Time: 30 minutes
Servings: 1
Ingredients:

- 2.5 oz. dry spinach
- 1/4 red bell pepper
- Artichoke (drain the liquid)
- Green onions
- Dried tomatoes
- Two eggs
- Italian seasoning
- Salt

- Pepper

Directions:
1. Preheat oven to medium heat. Brush a bit of oil on the cast-iron skillet.
2. Mix all the vegetables and add some seasoning.
3. Spread the vegetables evenly in the pan.
4. Whisk the eggs and add some milk. Add some salt and pepper.
5. Mix in some cheese (helps to make it fluffier).
6. Pour the egg mixture in the saucepan. Place the pan inside the oven for about 30 minutes. Enjoy!

CHOCOLATE SWEET POTATO PUDDING

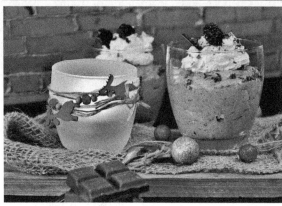

Preparation Time: 5 minutes
Cooking Time: 2 minutes
Servings: 1
Ingredients:
- 2 well-cooked sweet potatoes
- 2 tablespoons cocoa powder
- 2 tablespoons maple syrup
- ¼ cups plant-based milk (for ex. almond milk)
- ¼ tablespoons salt
- ¼ tablespoons vanilla extract

Directions:
1. Inside the food processor, put all the ingredients.
2. Blend thoroughly for about 30 seconds to 1 minute. Voilà!

PEANUT BUTTER AND PROTEIN PANCAKE

Preparation Time: 10 minutes
Cooking Time: 15 minutes
Servings: 1
Ingredients:
- ½ cup oat flour
- ½ cup gluten-free chocolate pancake mix
- ½ cup almond milk
- 1 egg
- 1 tablespoon coconut water
- 1 tablespoon peanut butter
- Fresh fruits slices

Directions:
1. Preheat a saucepan to medium heat.
2. Mix the flour and the pancake mix in a mixing bowl. Mix the almond milk and eggs with coconut water in another bowl. Mix the dry and wet ingredients thoroughly to form a delicate batter.
3. Spray the preheated saucepan with some coconut oil.
4. Put the batter into the saucepan with a measuring cup and allow it to cook for a few minutes.
5. Allow to cool and top with peanut butter and fresh fruit slices.

ZUCCHINI FRITTATA

Preparation Time: 20 minutes
Cooking Time: 20 minutes
Servings: 1
Ingredients:
- 2 large zucchinis
- 1½ teaspoon of salt
- 2 eggs

- ½ cup chopped green onions
- 1 cup flour
- ½ teaspoon of black pepper
- 1 teaspoon of baking powder
- 2 tablespoons of oil

Directions:

1. Wash the two zucchinis.
2. Cut off the zucchinis on its ends and grate them in a large mixing bowl.
3. Stir in 1 teaspoon of salt and set aside for about 10 minutes (The salt helps to draw out the water from the zucchinis). Squeeze dry the grated zucchinis to remove as much water as possible.
4. Then followed by the two whole eggs and the chopped green onions.
5. In a bowl, mix a cup flour, ½ teaspoon of salt, ½ teaspoon of black pepper, and one teaspoon of baking powder.
6. Next, pour the contents of the smaller bowl to those of the larger bowl containing the grated zucchinis.
7. Stir them all together and make sure they are well mixed.
8. Preheat a saucepan to medium temperature and add two tablespoons of oil.
9. Add the zucchini mixture a heaping tablespoonful at a time. Sauté the mixture for about 4 minutes on each side, to achieve a golden-brown color. Add more oil to the pan if needed. Serve and enjoy!

TEX-MEX TOFU BREAKFAST TACOS

Preparation Time: 10 minutes
Cooking Time: 15 minutes
Servings: 1
Ingredients:

- 8 oz. firm tofu
- 1 cup well-cooked black bean
- 1/4 red onion
- 1 cup fresh coriander
- 1 ripe avocado
- 1/2 cup salsa
- 1 medium-sized lime
- 5 whole corn tortillas
- 1/2 teaspoon garlic powder
- 1/2 teaspoon chili powder
- 1/8 teaspoon of sea salt
- 1 tablespoon salsa
- 1 tablespoon water

Directions:

1. Dice the red onions, avocados, coriander, and keep in separate bowls.
2. Also, slice the limes and keep in individual bowls. Wrap the tofu and place under a cast-iron skillet.
3. In the meantime, heat a saucepan to medium heat and cook the black beans, add a little amount of salt, cumin, and chili powder. Then decrease the heat to a low simmer and set aside.
4. Add the tofu spices and salsa into a bowl, then add some water and set aside.
5. Heat another skillet to medium heat. Pour some oil into the skillet, and then crumble the tofu into it.
6. Stir-fry for about 5 minutes until the tofu begins to brown. Add some seasoning and continue to cook for about 5 to 10 minutes, and then set aside. Heat the tortillas in oven to 250°F.
7. Top the tortillas with tofu scramble, avocado, salsa, coriander, black beans, and lime juice. Serve immediately.

MOCHA OATMEAL

Preparation Time: 5 minutes
Cooking Time: 10 minutes
Servings: 1
Ingredients:

- 1 banana
- ½ cup oats
- 1 cup coffee
- ¼ teaspoon salt
- 1 teaspoon walnut
- ½ teaspoon cacao powder
- 1 cup milk
- Honey

Directions:

1. Preheat a saucepan to medium heat. Put the oats in a saucepan.

2. Slice the banana, mash them, and add them to the oats. Add coffee, walnuts, cacao powder, and salt.
3. Stir and you may want to wait for it to simmer, practically until the mixture becomes sticky inconsistency.
4. Serve in a bowl and add milk and honey as desired. Enjoy!

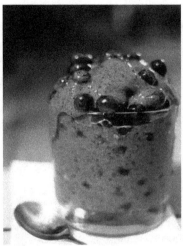

BLACK AND BLUEBERRY PROTEIN SMOOTHIE

Preparation Time: 5 minutes
Cooking Time: 0 minutes
Servings: 1
Ingredients:
- 1 cup sugar-free coconut milk (or any other plant-based milk of your choice)
- 1 scoop vanilla or natural protein powder
- 6 oz. fat-free vanilla Greek yogurt
- 2 tablespoons of milled flaxseed
- 1 cup berries (black or blue)
- 1 cup ice

Directions:
1. In the food processor, place all the ingredients.
2. Blend until smooth.
3. Pour into a cup and enjoy.

SHAKE CAKE FUELING

Preparation Time: 5 minutes
Cooking Time: 0 minutes
Servings: 1
Ingredients:
- 1 packet Protein shakes.
- ¼ teaspoon baking powder
- 2 tablespoons eggbeaters or egg whites
- 2 tablespoons water.

Directions:
1. Begin by preheating the oven.
2. Mix all the ingredients begin with the dry ingredients first before adding the wet ingredients.
3. After the mixture/batter is ready, pour gently into muffin cups.
4. Inside the oven, place, and bake for about 16–18minutes or until it is baked and ready. Allow it to cool completely. Add additional toppings of your choice and ensure your delicious shake cake is refreshing.

LEAN AND GREEN SMOOTHIE 1

Preparation Time: 5 minutes
Cooking Time: 0 minutes
Servings: 1
Ingredients:
- 2 ½ cups of kale leaves
- ¾ cup chilled apple juice
- 1 cup cubed pineapple
- ½ cup frozen green grapes
- ½ cup chopped apple

Directions:
1. Place the pineapple, apple juice, apple, frozen seedless grapes, and kale leaves in a blender.
2. Cover and blend until it's smooth.
3. Smoothie is ready and can be garnished with halved grapes if you wish.

LEAN AND GREEN SMOOTHIE 2

Preparation Time: 5 minutes

Cooking Time: 0 minutes

Servings: 1

Ingredients:

- 6 kale leaves
- 2 peeled oranges
- 2 cups mango kombucha
- 2 cups chopped pineapple
- 2 cups water

Directions:

1. Break up the oranges, place in the blender.
2. Add the mango kombucha, chopped pineapple, and kale leaves into the blender.
3. Blend everything until it is smooth. Smoothie is ready to be taken.

TROPICAL GREENS SMOOTHIE

Preparation Time: 5 Minutes

Cooking Time: 0 Minutes

Servings: 1

Ingredients:

- 1/2 large navel orange, peeled and segmented
- 1 banana
- 1/2 cup frozen mango chunks
- 1 cup frozen spinach
- 1 celery stalk, broken into pieces
- 1 tablespoon cashew butter or almond butter
- 1/2 tablespoon spiraling
- 1/2 tablespoon ground flaxseed
- 1/2 cup unsweetened nondairy milk
- Water, for thinning (optional)

Directions:

1. In a high-speed blender or food processor, combine the bananas, orange, mango, spinach, celery, cashew butter, spiraling (if using), flaxseed, and milk.
2. Blend until creamy, adding more milk or water to thin the smoothie if too thick. Serve immediately!

VITAMIN C SMOOTHIE CUBES

Preparation Time: 5 minutes

Cooking Time: 8 hours to chill

Servings: 1

Ingredients:

- 1/8 large papaya
- 1/8 mango
- 1/4 cups chopped pineapple, fresh or frozen
- 1/8 cup raw cauliflower florets, fresh or frozen
- 1/4 large navel oranges, peeled and halved
- 1/4 large orange bell pepper stemmed, seeded, and coarsely chopped

Directions:

1. Halve the papaya and mango, remove the pits, and scoop their soft flesh into a high-speed blender.
2. Add the pineapple, cauliflower, oranges, and bell pepper. Blend until smooth.
3. Evenly divide the puree between 2 (16-compartment) ice cube trays and place them on a level surface in your freezer. Freeze for at least 8 hours.
4. The cubes can be left in the ice cube trays until use or transferred to a freezer bag. The frozen cubes are good for about three weeks in a standard freezer or up to 6 months in a chest freezer.

OVERNIGHT CHOCOLATE CHIA PUDDING

Preparation Time: 2 minutes

Cooking Time: Overnight to Chill

Servings: 1

Ingredients:

- 1/8 cup chia seeds
- 1/2 cup unsweetened nondairy milk
- 1 tablespoon raw cacao powder

- 1/2 teaspoon vanilla extract
- 1/2 teaspoon pure maple syrup

Directions:

1. Stir together the chia seeds, milk, cacao powder, vanilla, and maple syrup in a large bowl. Divide between 2 (½-pint) covered glass jars or containers. Refrigerate overnight. Stir before serving.

SLOW COOKER SAVORY BUTTERNUT SQUASH OATMEAL

Preparation Time: 15 minutes
Cooking Time: 6 to 8 hours
Servings: 1
Ingredients:

- 1/4 cup steel-cut oats
- 1/2 cups cubed (½-inch pieces) peeled butternut squash
- 3/4 cups water
- 1/16 cup unsweetened nondairy milk
- 1/4 tablespoon chia seed
- 1/2 teaspoons yellow (mellow) miso paste
- 3/4 teaspoons ground ginger
- 1/4 tablespoon sesame seed, toasted
- 1/4 tablespoon chopped scallion, green parts only
- Shredded carrot, for serving (optional)

Directions:

1. In a slow cooker, combine the oats, butternut squash, and water. Cover the slow cooker and cook on low for 6 to 8 hours, or until the squash is fork-tender. Using a potato masher or heavy spoon, roughly mash the cooked butternut squash. Stir to combine with the oats.
2. Whisk together the milk, chia seeds, miso paste, and ginger to combine in a large bowl. Stir the mixture into the oats. Top your oatmeal bowl with sesame seeds and scallion for more plant-based fiber, top with shredded carrot.

CARROT CAKE OATMEAL

Preparation Time: 10 minutes
Cooking Time: 15 minutes
Servings: 1
Ingredients:

- 1/8 cup pecans
- 1/2 cup finely shredded carrot
- 1/4 cup old-fashioned oats
- 5/8 cups unsweetened nondairy milk
- 1/2 tablespoon pure maple syrup
- 1/2 teaspoon ground cinnamon
- 1/2 teaspoon ground ginger
- 1/8 teaspoon ground nutmeg
- 1 tablespoon chia seed

Directions:

1. Over medium-high heat in a skillet, toast the pecans for 3 to 4 minutes, often stirring, until browned and fragrant (watch closely, as they can burn quickly). Pour the pecans onto a cutting board and coarsely chop them. Set aside.
2. In an 8-quart pot over medium-high heat, combine the carrot, oats, milk, maple syrup, cinnamon, ginger, and nutmeg. When it is already boiling, reduce the heat to medium-low. Cook, uncovered, for 10 minutes, stirring occasionally. Stir in the chopped pecans and chia seeds. Serve immediately.

SPICED SORGHUM AND BERRIES

Preparation Time: 5 minutes
Cooking Time: 1 hour
Servings: 1
Ingredients:

- 1/4 cup whole-grain sorghum
- 1/4 teaspoon ground cinnamon
- 1/4 teaspoon Chinese five-spice powder
- 3/4 cups water
- 1/4 cup unsweetened nondairy milk
- 1/4 teaspoon vanilla extract
- 1/2 tablespoons pure maple syrup
- 1/2 tablespoon chia seed
- 1/8 cup sliced almonds
- 2 cups fresh raspberries, divided

Directions:

1. Using a large pot over medium-high heat, stir together the sorghum, cinnamon, five-spice powder, and water. Wait for the water to a boil, cover the bank, and reduce the heat to medium-low. Cook for 1 hour, or until the sorghum is soft and chewy. If the sorghum grains are still hard, add another cup of water and cook for 15 minutes more. Using a glass measuring cup, whisk together the milk, vanilla, and maple syrup to blend. Add the mixture to the sorghum and the chia seeds, almonds, and 1 cup of raspberries. Gently stir to combine.

2. When serving, top with the remaining 1 cup of fresh raspberries.

RAW-CINNAMON-APPLE NUT BOWL

Preparation Time: 15 minutes

Cooking Time: 1 hour to chill

Servings: 1

Ingredients:

- 1 green apple halved, seeded, and cored
- 3/4 honey crisp apples, halved, seeded, and cored
- 1/4 teaspoon freshly squeezed lemon juice
- 1 pitted Medrol dates
- 1/8 teaspoon ground cinnamon
- Pinch ground nutmeg
- 1/2 tablespoons chia seeds, plus more for serving (optional)
- 1/4 tablespoon hemp seed
- 1/8 cup chopped walnuts
- Nut butter, for serving (optional)

Directions:

1. Finely dice half the green apple and honey crisp apple. With the lemon juice, store it in an airtight container while you work on the next steps. Coarsely chop the remaining apples and the dates. Transfer to a food processor and add the cinnamon and nutmeg. Check it several times if it combines, then processes for 2 to 3 minutes to puree. Stir the puree into the reserved diced apples. Stir in the chia seeds (if using), hemp seeds, and walnuts. Chill for at least 1 hour. Enjoy! Serve as is or top with additional chia seeds and nut butter (if using).

PEANUT BUTTER AND CACAO BREAKFAST QUINOA

Preparation Time: 5 minutes

Cooking Time: 10 minutes

Servings: 1

Ingredients:

- 1/3 cup quinoa flakes
- 1/2 cup unsweetened nondairy milk
- 1/2 cup water
- 1/8 cup raw cacao powder
- 1 tablespoon natural creamy peanut butter
- 1/8 teaspoon ground cinnamon
- 1 banana, mashed
- Fresh berries of choice, for serving
- Chopped nuts of choice, for serving

Directions:

1. Using an 8-quart pot over medium-high heat, stir together the quinoa flakes, milk, water, cacao powder, peanut butter, and cinnamon. Cook and stir it until the mixture begins to simmer. Turn the heat to medium-low and cook for 3 to 5 minutes, stirring frequently.

2. Stir in the bananas and cook until hot. Serve topped with fresh berries, nuts, and a splash of milk.

VANILLA BUCKWHEAT PORRIDGE

Preparation Time: 5 minutes

Cooking Time: 25 minutes

Servings: 1

Ingredients:

- 1 cup water
- 1/4 cup raw buckwheat grouts
- 1/4 teaspoon ground cinnamon
- 1/4 banana, sliced
- 1/16 cup golden raisins
- 1/16 cup dried currants
- 1/16 cup sunflower seeds

18

- 1/2 tablespoons chia seeds
- 1/4 tablespoon hemp seed
- 1/4 tablespoon sesame seed, toasted
- 1/8 cup unsweetened nondairy milk
- 1/4 tablespoon pure maple syrup
- 1/4 teaspoon vanilla extract

Directions:

1. Boil the water in a pot. Stir in the buckwheat, cinnamon, and banana. Cook the mixture. Mixing it and wait for it to boil, then reduce the heat to medium-low. Cover the pot and cook for 15 minutes, or until the buckwheat is tender. Remove from the heat. Stir in the raisins, currants, sunflower seeds, chia seeds, hemp seeds, sesame seeds, milk, maple syrup, and vanilla. Cover the pot. Wait for 10 minutes before serving. Serve as is or top as desired.

BEST WHOLE WHEAT PANCAKES

Preparation Time: 10 minutes
Cooking Time: 20 minutes
Servings: 1
Ingredients:

- 3/4 tablespoons ground flaxseed
- 2 tablespoons warm water
- 1/2 cups whole wheat pastry flour
- 1/8 cup rye flour
- 1/2 tablespoons double-acting baking powder
- 1/4 teaspoon ground cinnamon
- 1/8 teaspoon ground ginger
- 1 cup unsweetened nondairy milk
- 3/4 tablespoons pure maple syrup
- 1/4 teaspoon vanilla extract

Directions:

1. Mix the warm water and flaxseed in a large bowl. Set aside for at least 5 minutes.
2. Whisk together the pastry and rye flours, baking powder, cinnamon, and ginger to combine.
3. Whisk together the milk, maple syrup, and vanilla in a large bowl. Make use of a spatula, fold the wet ingredients into the dry ingredients. Fold in the soaked flaxseed until fully incorporated.
4. Heat a large skillet or nonstick griddle over medium-high heat. Working in batches, 3 to 4 pancakes at a time, add ¼-cup portions of batter to the hot skillet. Until golden brown, cook for 3 to 4 minutes each side or no liquid batter is visible.

SPICED PUMPKIN MUFFINS

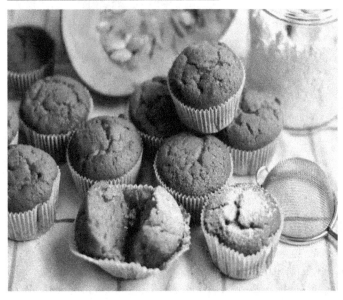

Servings: 1   **Cooking Time:** 20 minutes
Ingredients: **Preparation Time:** 15 minutes

- 1/6 tablespoons ground flaxseed
- 1/24 cup water
- 1/8 cups whole wheat flour
- 1/6 teaspoons baking powder
- 5/6 teaspoons ground cinnamon
- 1/12 teaspoon baking soda
- 1/12 teaspoon ground ginger
- 1/16 teaspoon ground nutmeg
- 1/32 teaspoon ground cloves
- 1/6 cup pumpkin puree
- 1/12 cup pure maple syrup
- 1/24 cup unsweetened applesauce
- 1/24 cup unsweetened nondairy milk
- 1/2 teaspoons vanilla extract

Directions:

1. Preheat the oven to 350°F. Line a 12-cup metal muffin pan with parchment paper liners or use a silicone muffin pan.
2. First, mix the flaxseed and water in a large bowl then keep it aside. In a medium bowl, stir together the flour, baking powder, cinnamon, baking soda, ginger, nutmeg, and cloves.
3. In a medium bowl, stir up the maple syrup, pumpkin puree, applesauce, milk, and vanilla. Crease the wet ingredients into the dry ingredients make use of a spatula. Fold the soaked flaxseed into the batter until evenly combined, but do not over mix the batter, or your muffins will become dense. Spoon about ¼ cup of batter per muffin into your prepared muffin pan. Bake for 18 to 20 minutes, or until a toothpick inserted into the center of a muffin comes out clean. Remove the muffins from the pan. Transfer to a wire rack for cooling. Store in an airtight container that is at room temperature.

ORANGE RESOLUTION SMOOTHIE

Preparation Time: 5 minutes
Cooking Time: 0 minutes
Servings: 1
Ingredients:

- 1/4 cup orange juice
- 1/2 cup Greek yogurt
- 1/2 cup frozen mango chunks
- 1 banana, peeled, frozen
- 1/4 cup miniature carrots
- 1/2 cup frozen peach slices
- 1 tablespoon honey
- 1/4 cup pineapple pieces

Directions:

1. Gather all the ingredients.
2. Start a high-powered blender, and then add together every ingredient into it in the order mentioned in the list.
3. Turn it on for 45 to 60 seconds or more reliant on the blender, until well blended and smooth, and then divide the smoothie between two glasses. Serve straight away.

SPICY CARROT, AVOCADO, AND TOMATO SMOOTHIE

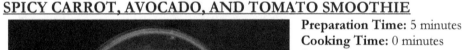

Preparation Time: 5 minutes
Cooking Time: 0 minutes
Servings: 1
Ingredients:

- 3/4 cup coconut water, unsweetened
- ½ a medium cucumber, unpeeled, chopped
- 1 medium tomato, deseeded, chopped
- 1 avocado, peeled, pitted
- 1 cup chopped romaine lettuce
- 1 medium carrot, peeled, diced
- 1 lime, peeled, halved
- 1 clove garlic, peeled
- 3/4 teaspoon sea salt
- 1/8 teaspoon cayenne pepper
- 1 tablespoon olive oil
- 1 cup ice cubes

Directions:

1. Gather all the ingredients. Add all the ingredients into it in the order cited in a blender.
2. Pulse for 45 to 60 seconds or more varying on the blender, up until well combined and smooth, and then distribute the smoothie amongst two glasses. Serve straight away.

ZUCCHINI BREAD SMOOTHIE

Preparation Time: 5 minutes
Cooking Time: 0 minutes
Servings: 1
Ingredients:

- 2 cups almond milk, unsweetened
- ½ cup baby spinach leaves, fresh, rinsed
- ½ cup rolled oats
- 2 cups chopped zucchini, fresh or frozen
- 1 teaspoon ground cinnamon
- 1 tablespoon maple syrup
- ¼ teaspoon ground nutmeg
- ¼ cup walnut halves
- 1 cup ice cubes

Directions:

1. Gather all the ingredients.
2. In a high-powered blender, add up all the ingredients into it in the sort cited in the list.
3. Turn it on for 45 to 60 seconds or further dependent on the blender, until well mixed and smooth, and then distribute the smoothie between two glasses.
4. Serve straight away.

CAULIFLOWER AND BLUEBERRY SMOOTHIE

Preparation Time: 5 minutes
Cooking Time: 0 minutes
Servings: 1
Ingredients:

- 1 cup Greek yogurt, unsweetened
- 2 tablespoons peanut butter
- 1 ¼ cup cauliflower florets, frozen
- 1 clementines, peeled
- ½ cup spinach leaves, rinsed
- 1 cup blueberries, frozen

Directions:

1. Gather all the ingredients.
2. Socket a high-powdered blender, and later combine all the components into it in the order mentioned in the ingredients list. Let it blend for 45 to 60 seconds or more reliant on the blender, until properly mixed and smooth. Then, divide the smoothie between two glasses. Serve straight away.

BUTTERNUT SQUASH SMOOTHIE

Preparation Time: 5 minutes
Cooking Time: 0 minutes
Servings: 1
Ingredients:

- 2 cups almond milk, unsweetened
- ½ cup water
- 1 cup butternut squash pieces, frozen
- 2 bananas, peeled, frozen
- 1 cup raspberries, frozen
- 2 tablespoons hemp seeds
- 1 tablespoons chia seeds
- 1 teaspoon ground cinnamon
- 1/4 cup peanut butter

Directions:

1. In a high-powdered blender, add all the ingredients into it in the order in the list.
2. Turn it on for 45 to 60 seconds or further differing on the blender, until perfectly combined and smooth, and then distribute the smoothie among two glasses. Serve up straight away.

AVOCADO AND KALE SUPER FOOD SMOOTHIE

Preparation Time: 5 minutes
Cooking Time: 0 minutes
Servings: 1
Ingredients:

- 1/2 cup almond milk, unsweetened

- 1/2 cup blueberry yogurt
- 1 banana, peeled, frozen
- 1/2 avocado, peeled, pitted
- 1 cup kale, stemmed, rinsed

Directions:
1. Gather all the ingredients.
2. Plug in a high-powered blender, and then add every one of the ingredients listed.
3. Turn it on for 45 to 60 seconds or extra dependent on the blender, until properly combined and smooth, and then divide the smoothie between two glasses. Serve straight away.

PINEAPPLE CELERY SMOOTHIE

Preparation Time: 5 minutes
Cooking Time: 0 minutes
Servings: 1
Ingredients:
- 1/4 cup almond milk, unsweetened
- 1/2 pear, cored, chopped
- 1 stalk celery, chopped
- 1/2 banana, peeled, frozen
- 1/2 teaspoon honey
- 1/2 cup pineapple pieces, cubed

Directions:
1. Gather all the ingredients.
2. Plug in a high-powdered blender, and then add all the ingredients into it in the order mentioned in the list.
3. Turn it on for 45 to 60 seconds or more depending on the blender, until well blended and smooth, and then distribute the smoothie between two glasses. Serve straight away.

MANGO AND CUCUMBER SMOOTHIE

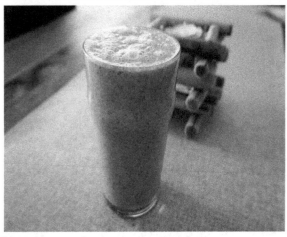

Preparation Time: 5 minutes
Cooking Time: 0 minutes
Servings: 1
Ingredients:
- 1 ½ cup coconut milk, unsweetened
- 4 teaspoons lime juice
- 1 cup baby spinach leaves, fresh, rinsed
- 2 cup mango pieces, fresh or frozen
- 4 mint leaves, rinsed
- 1 cup chopped cucumber, deseeded, peeled
- 1/4 teaspoon cayenne pepper
- 1 cup ice cubes

Directions:
1. Collect all the ingredients.
2. Plug in a high-powered blender and all the ingredients into it in the directive mentioned in the list.
3. Pulse for 45 to 60 seconds or extra depending on the blender, up until well combined and smooth, and then distribute the smoothie between two glasses. Serve straight away.

MELON, KALE, AND BROCCOLI SMOOTHIE

Preparation Time: 5 minutes
Cooking Time: 0 minutes
Servings: 1
Ingredients:
- 2 cups coconut water, unsweetened
- 2/3 cup broccoli florets
- 2 cups honeydew melon pieces

- 1 lime, peeled, deseeded, halved
- ½ cup kale, stemmed, rinsed
- 2 Medrol dates pitted
- ½ cup mint leaves
- 1 cup ice cubes

Directions:
1. Gather all the ingredients.
2. Plug in a high-powered blender, and then add all the ingredients in the order indicated in the list.
3. Pulse for 45 to 60 seconds or extra diverging on the blender, until well mixed and smooth out, and then distribute the smoothie between two glasses. Serve straight away.

AVOCADO AND CUCUMBER SMOOTHIE

Preparation Time: 5 minutes

Cooking Time: 0 minutes

Servings: 1

Ingredients:

- 1 cup water, chilled
- 1 large cucumber, deseeded
- 1 avocado, cored, peeled

Directions:
1. Gather all the ingredients.
2. Plug in a high-powered blender, then combine all the ingredients into it in the order mentioned in the register.
3. Thump for 45 to 60 seconds or more dependent on the blender, until nicely combined and smooth, and then divide the smoothie between two glasses. Serve straight away.

APPLE, BANANA, AND COLLARD GREENS SMOOTHIE

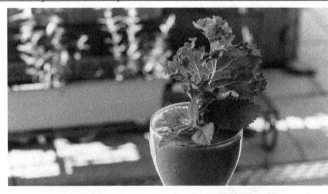

Preparation Time: 5 minutes

Cooking Time: 0 minutes

Servings: 1

Ingredients:

- 1 cup water, chilled
- 2 green apples, cored
- 1 large banana, peeled, frozen
- 1 ½ cup collard greens, frozen

Directions:
1. Gather all the ingredients.
2. Plug in a high-powdered blender, and then combine the whole ingredients into it in the directive mentioned in the list. Pulse for 45 to 60 seconds or more varying on the blender, until well blended and smooth, and then allocate the smoothie between two glasses. Serve straight away.

BROCCOLI AND ORANGE SMOOTHIE

Preparation Time: 5 minutes

Servings: 1

Ingredients:

- 1 cup water, chilled
- 2 broccoli heads
- 1 orange, peeled

Directions:
1. Gather all the ingredients.
2. Plug in a high-powered blender, and later add every ingredient into it in the order stated in the list.
3. Pulse for 45 to 60 seconds or more depending on the blender, until well combined and smooth, then distributing the smoothie between two glasses. Serve straight away.

SWEET KIWI AND MINT SMOOTHIE

Preparation Time: 5 minutes

Cooking Time: 0 minutes

Servings: 1

Ingredients:
- 1 cup water, chilled
- 2 kiwis, peeled
- 1 medium lemon, peeled
- ¼ cup mint leaves
- ¼ cup parsley leaves
- 2 teaspoons honey

Directions:
1. Gather all the ingredients.
2. Plug in a high-powered blender, and subsequently add all the ingredients into it in the order mentioned in the list.
3. Pulse for 45 to 60 seconds or extra differing on the blender, until perfectly combined and smooth out, and then divide the smoothie between two glasses. Serve straight away.

CUCUMBER, CELERY, AND APPLE SMOOTHIE

Preparation Time: 5 minutes

Cooking Time: 0 minutes

Servings: 1

Ingredients:
- 1/2 cup water, chilled
- 1/4 lemon, juiced
- 1/2 large stalk of celery
- 1 medium green apple, cored
- 1/2 large cucumber

Directions:
1. Gather all the ingredients.
2. Plug in a high-powdered blender, and then add all the ingredients into it in the order indicated in the list.
3. Turn it on for 45 to 60 seconds or more differing on the blender, until properly combined and smooth, and then distribute the smoothie between two glasses. Serve straight away.

Tea with Coconut

Preparation Time: 10 minutes

Cooking Time: 0 minutes;

Servings: 2

Ingredients:
- 2 tea bags, cinnamon-flavored
- 2 tbsp MCT oil
- ¼ cup coconut milk, unsweetened
- 2 cups boiling water

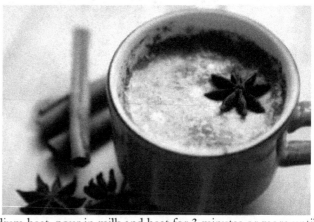

Directions:
1. Pour boiling water between two mugs, add a tea into each mug and let them steep for 5 minutes.
2. Meanwhile, take a small saucepan, place it over medium heat, pour in milk and heat for 3 minutes or more until hot.
3. After 5 minutes, remove tea bags from mugs, stir in milk, and MCT oil by using a milk frother until combined and then serve.

Special Lunch Recipes

Bacon Spaghetti Squash Carbonara

Preparation Time: 20 minutes

Cooking Time: 40 minutes

Servings: 4

Ingredients:

- 1 small spaghetti squash
- 6 ounces' bacon (roughly chopped)
- 1 large tomato (sliced)
- 2 chives (chopped)
- 1 garlic clove (minced)
- 6 ounces' low-fat cottage cheese
- 1 cup Gouda cheese (grated)
- 2 tablespoons olive oil
- Salt and pepper, to taste

Directions:

1. Preheat the oven to 350°F.
2. Cut the squash spaghetti in half, brush with some olive oil and bake for 20–30 minutes, skin side up. Remove from the oven and remove the core with a fork, creating the spaghetti.
3. Heat one tablespoon of olive oil in a skillet. Cook the bacon for about 1 minute until crispy.
4. Quickly wipe out the pan with paper towels.
5. Heat another tablespoon of oil and sauté the garlic, tomato and chives for 2–3 minutes. Add the spaghetti and sauté for another 5 minutes, stirring occasionally to keep from burning. Begin to add the cottage cheese, about 2 tablespoons at a time. If the sauce becomes thicken, add about a cup of water. The sauce should be creamy, but not too runny or thick. Allow to cook for another 3 minutes. Serve immediately.

Cauliflower Crust Pizza

Preparation Time: 15 minutes

Cooking Time: 30–35 minutes

Servings: 1

Ingredients:

- 1/4 cauliflower (it should be cut into smaller portions)
- 1/16 grated parmesan cheese
- 1/2 egg
- ½ teaspoon Italian seasoning
- 1/16 teaspoon kosher salt
- 1 cups of freshly grated mozzarella
- 1/4 cup spicy pizza sauce.
- Basil leaves, for garnishing.

Directions:

1. Begin by preheating your oven while using the parchment paper to rim the baking sheet.
2. Process the cauliflower into a fine powder, and then transfer to a bowl before putting it into the microwave. Leave for about 5–6 minutes to get it soft.
3. Transfer the microwaved cauliflower to a clean and dry kitchen towel. Leave it to cool.
4. When cold, use the kitchen towel to wrap the cauliflower and then get rid of all the moisture by wringing the towel. Continue squeezing until water is gone completely.
5. Put the cauliflower, Italian seasoning, parmesan, egg, salt, and mozzarella (1 cup). Stir very well until well combined. Transfer the combined mixture to the baking sheet previously prepared, pressing it into a 10-inch round shape. Wait for it to bake until it becomes golden in color.
6. Take the baked crust out of the oven and use the spicy pizza sauce and mozzarella (the leftover 1 cup) to top it. Put it again inside the oven for ten more minutes until the cheese melts and looks bubbly.
7. Garnish using fresh basil leaves. You can also enjoy this with salad.

Delicious Pizza

Preparation Time: 5–10 minutes

Cooking Time: 15–20 minutes

Servings: 1

Ingredients:

- 1/4 cup mashed potato
- 1/2 egg whites
- 1/4 tablespoon baking powder
- 3/4 oz. reduced-fat shredded mozzarella
- 1/8 cup sliced white mushrooms
- 1/16 cup pizza sauce
- 3/4 oz. ground beef
- 1/4 sliced black olives
- You also need a sauté pan, baking sheets, and parchment paper

Directions:

1. Preheat the oven to 400°F.
2. Mix your baking powder and garlic potato packet. Add egg whites to your mixture and stir well until it blends.
3. Line the baking sheet with parchment paper and pour the mixed batter onto it.
4. Put another parchment paper on top of the batter and spread out the batter to a 1/8-inch circle.
5. Then place another baking sheet on top; this way, the matter is between two baking sheets.
6. Place into an oven and bake for about 8 minutes until the pizza crust is golden brown.
7. For the toppings, place your ground beef in a sauté pan and fry until its brown and wash your mushrooms very well.
8. After the crust is baked, remove the top layer of parchment paper carefully to prevent the paper from sticking to the pizza crust. Put your toppings on top of the crust and bake for an extra 8 minutes.
9. Once ready, slide the pizza off the parchment paper and into a plate.

Mini Mac in a Bowl

Preparation Time: 5 minutes

Cooking Time: 15 minutes

Servings: 1

Ingredients:

- 5 oz. lean ground beef
- 2 tablespoons diced white or yellow onion.
- 1/8 teaspoon onion powder
- 1/8 teaspoon white vinegar
- 1 oz. dill pickle slices
- 1 teaspoon sesame seed
- 3 cups shredded romaine lettuce
- Cooking spray
- 2 tablespoons reduced-fat shredded cheddar cheese
- 2 tablespoons wish-bone light thousand island as dressing

Directions:

1. Place a lightly greased small skillet on fire to heat.
2. Add your onion to cook for about 2–3 minutes.
3. Next, add the beef and allow it to cook until it is brown.
4. Next, mix your vinegar and onion powder with the dressing.
5. Finally, top the lettuce with the cooked meat and sprinkle cheese on it, add your pickle slices.
6. Drizzle the mixture with the sauce and sprinkle the sesame seeds also. Enjoy!

Lean and Green Chicken Pesto Pasta

Preparation Time: 5 minutes

Cooking Time: 15 minutes

Servings: 1

Ingredients:

- 3 cups raw kale leaves
- 2 tablespoon olive oil
- 2 cups fresh basil
- ¼ teaspoon salt

- 3 tablespoon lemon juice
- 3 garlic cloves
- 2 cups cooked chicken breast
- 1 cup baby spinach

- 6 oz. uncooked chicken pasta
- 3 oz. diced fresh mozzarella
- Basil leaves or red pepper flakes to garnish

Directions:

1. Start by making the pesto, add the kale, lemon juice, basil, garlic cloves, olive oil, and salt to a blender and blend until it is smooth.
2. Add pepper to taste.
3. Cook the pasta and strain off the water. Reserve ¼ cup of the liquid.
4. Get a bowl and mix everything, the cooked pasta, pesto, diced chicken, spinach, mozzarella, and the reserved pasta liquid. Sprinkle the mixture with additional chopped basil or red paper flakes (optional). Enjoy!

Polenta with Seared Pears

Preparation Time: 10 minutes
Cooking Time: 50 minutes
Servings: 1
Ingredients:

- 1 cup water, divided, plus more as needed
- 1/2 cups coarse cornmeal
- 1 tablespoon pure maple syrup
- 1/4 tablespoon molasses
- 1/4 teaspoon ground cinnamon
- 1/2 ripe pears, cored and diced
- 1/4 cup fresh cranberries
- 1/4 teaspoon chopped fresh rosemary leaves

Directions:

1. In a pan, cook 5 cups of water to a simmer. While whisking continuously to avoid clumping, slowly pour in the cornmeal. Cook, often stirring with a heavy spoon, for 30 minutes. The polenta should be thick and creamy. While the polenta cooks, in a saucepan over medium heat, stir together the maple syrup, molasses, the remaining ¼-cup of water, and the cinnamon until combined. Bring it to a simmer. Add the pears and cranberries. Cook for 10 minutes, occasionally stirring, until the pears are tender and start to brown. Remove from the heat. Stir in the rosemary and let the mixture sit for 5 minutes. If it is too thick, add another ¼ cup of water and return to the heat. Top with the cranberry-pear mixture.

Bacon and Cauliflower Mac and Cheese

Preparation Time: 5 minutes
Cooking Time: 20 minutes
Servings: 2
Ingredients:

- 2 strips of bacon
- ½ cup cauliflower florets, chopped
- 3 tablespoons butter, unsalted
- 3 ounces whipped topping
- 3 tablespoons grated cheddar cheese

EXTRA:

- ½ teaspoon salt
- 1/8 teaspoon ground black pepper
- ¼ teaspoon cayenne pepper
- ¾ cup of water

Directions:

1. Take a skillet pan, place it over medium heat and when hot, add bacon and cook for 5 minutes or until crispy.
2. Transfer bacon to a plate, pat dry with paper towels, chop the bacon and set aside until required.
3. When done, drain the cauliflower and then set aside until required.
4. Return saucepan over medium heat, add butter, whipped topping, salt, black pepper, and cayenne pepper, cook for 3 to 5 minutes until the butter has melted and a thick sauce comes together, stirring continuously.
5. Add bacon into the sauce, stir until combined, and remove the pan from heat.
6. Serve straight away.

Taco Stuffed Avocados

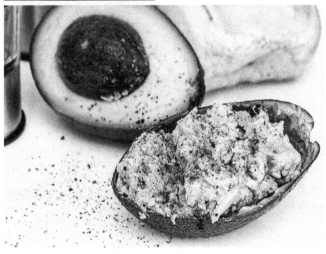

Preparation Time: 5 minutes
Cooking Time: 12 minutes
Servings: 1
Ingredients:

- ¼ pound ground turkey
- 2-ounce tomato sauce
- 1 medium avocado, pitted, halved
- ½ cup shredded cheddar cheese
- 2 tablespoon shredded lettuce

EXTRA:

- 1/8 teaspoon garlic powder
- ¼ teaspoon salt
- ½ tablespoon red chili powder

Directions:

1. Take a skillet pan, place it over medium heat, add ground turkey and cook for 5 minutes until nicely golden brown. Reserve the grease for later use, then season the turkey with garlic powder, salt, and red chili powder, stir in tomato sauce and cook for 3 minutes until the meat has thoroughly cooked.
2. Cut the avocado into half, remove its pit and then stuff the crater with prepared meat.
3. Top meat with cheddar cheese and lettuce and serve.

Tuna Cakes

Preparation Time: 5 minutes
Cooking Time: 6 minutes
Servings: 2
Ingredients:

- 5-ounce tuna, packed in water
- 1 tablespoon mustard
- 1 teaspoon garlic powder
- 1 tablespoon coconut oil

EXTRA:

- ¼ teaspoon salt
- 1/8 teaspoon ground black pepper

Directions:

1. Drain the tuna, add it in a medium bowl and break it well with a fork.
2. Then add remaining ingredients, stir until well mixed and then shape the mixture into four patties.
3. Take a medium skillet pan, place it over medium heat, add oil and when hot, add tuna patties and cook for 3 minutes per side until golden brown. Serve patties straight away or serve as a wrap with iceberg lettuce.

Roasted Green Beans

Preparation Time: 5 minutes
Cooking Time: 25 minutes
Servings: 2
Ingredients:

- ½ pound green beans
- ½ cup grated parmesan cheese
- 3 tablespoons coconut oil
- ½ teaspoon garlic powder

EXTRA:

- 1/3 teaspoon salt
- 1/8 teaspoon ground black pepper

Directions:

1. Switch on the oven, then set it to 425 degrees F, and let preheat.

2. Take a baking sheet, line green beans on it, and set aside until required.
3. Prepare the dressing, and for this, place remaining ingredients in a bowl, except for cheese and whisk until combined. Drizzle the dressing over green beans, toss until well coated, and then bake for 20 minutes until green beans are tender-crisp.
4. Then sprinkle cheese on top of beans and continue roasting for 3 to 5 minutes or until cheese melts and nicely golden brown. Serve straight away.

Vegan Alfredo Fettuccine Pasta

Preparation Time: 15 minutes
Cooking Time: 15 minutes
Servings: 1
Ingredients:

- White potatoes - 2 medium
- White onion - ¼
- Italian seasoning - 1 tablespoon
- Lemon juice - 1 teaspoon
- Garlic - 2 cloves
- Salt - 1 teaspoon
- Fettuccine pasta - 12 ounces
- Raw cashew - ½ cup
- Nutritional yeast (optional) - 1 teaspoon
- Truffle oil (optional) - ¼ teaspoon

Directions:

1. Start by placing a pot on high flame and boiling 4 cups of water.
2. Peel the potatoes and cut them into small cubes. Cut the onion into cubes as well.
3. Add the potatoes and onions to the boiling water and cook for about 10 minutes.
4. Remove the onions and potatoes. Keep aside. Save the water.
5. Take another pot and fill it with water. Season generously with salt.
6. Toss in the fettuccine pasta and cook as per package instructions.
7. Take a blender and add in the raw cashews, veggies, nutritional yeast, truffle oil, lemon juice, and 1 cup of the saved water. Blend into a smooth puree. Add in the garlic and salt.
8. Drain the cooked pasta using a colander. Transfer into a mixing bowl.
9. Pour the prepared sauce on top of the cooked fettuccine pasta. Serve.

Spinach Pasta in Pesto Sauce

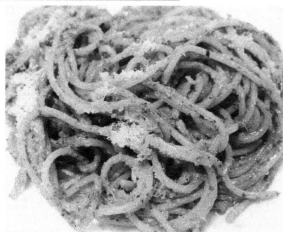

Preparation Time: 20 minutes
Cooking Time: 15 minutes
Servings: 1
Ingredients:

- Olive oil - 1 tablespoon
- Spinach - 5 ounces
- All-purpose flour - 2 cups
- Salt - 1 tablespoon plus ¼ teaspoon (keep it divided)
- Water - 2 tablespoons
- Roasted vegetable for serving
- Pesto for serving
- Fresh basil for serving

Directions:

1. Take a large pot and fill it with water. Place it over a high flame and bring the water to a boil. Add one tablespoon of salt. While the water is boiling, place a large saucepan over medium flame.
2. Pour in the olive oil and heat it through, toss in the spinach and sauté for 5 minutes.

3. Take a food processor and transfer the wilted spinach. Process until the spinach is fine in texture.
4. Add in the flour bit by bit and continue to process to form a crumbly dough.
5. Further, add ¼ teaspoon of salt and 1 tbsp of water while processing to bring the dough together. Add the remaining 1 tbsp of water if required.
6. Remove the dough onto a flat surface and sprinkle with flour. Knead well to form a dough ball.
7. Use a rolling pin to roll out the dough. The dimensions of the rolled dough should be 18 inches long and 12 inches wide. The thickness should be about ¼ - inch thick.
8. Cut the rolled dough into long and even strips using a pizza cutter. Make sure the strips are ½ - inch wide.
9. The strips need to be rolled into evenly sized thick noodles.
10. Toss in the prepared noodles and cook for about 4 minutes. Drain using a colander.
11. Transfer the noodles into a large mixing bowl and add in the roasted vegetables, pesto. Toss well to combine.
12. Garnish with basil leaves.

Shredded Chicken in a lettuce wrap

Preparation Time: 5 minutes
Cooking Time: 15 minutes
Servings: 2
Ingredients:

- 2 leaves of iceberg lettuce
- 2 large chicken thighs
- 2 tablespoon shredded cheddar cheese
- 3 cups hot water
- 4 tablespoon tomato sauce

EXTRA:

- 1 tablespoon soy sauce
- 1 tablespoon red chili powder
- ¾ teaspoon salt
- ½ teaspoon cracked black pepper

Directions:

1. Switch on the instant pot, place chicken thighs in it, and add remaining ingredients except for lettuce.
2. Stir until just mixed, shut the instant pot with a lid and cook for 15 minutes at high pressure and when done, release the stress naturally.
3. Then open the instant pot, transfer chicken to a cutting board and shred with two forks.
4. Evenly divide the chicken between two lettuce leaves, and drizzle with some of the cooking liquid, reserving the remaining cooking liquid for later use as chicken broth. Serve straight away.

Turkey Lettuce Wraps

Preparation Time: 5 minutes
Cooking Time: 15 minutes
Servings: 2
Ingredients:

- ¼ pound ground turkey
- 2 leaves of iceberg lettuce
- 1 tablespoon sesame oil
- 2 tablespoons soy sauce
- 1 tbsp cheddar cheese

EXTRA:

- 1 teaspoon garlic powder
- 1 teaspoon coconut oil
- ¼ teaspoon salt
- ¼ teaspoon cracked black pepper

Directions:

1. Take a skillet pan, place it over medium heat, add coconut oil and when hot, add turkey and cook for 7 to 10 minutes until nicely browned.
2. Meanwhile, rinse the lettuce leaves and pat dry with a paper towel, set aside until required. Prepare the sauce, and for this, whisk together sesame oil, soy sauce, garlic powder, salt, and black pepper. Pour the sauce into the cooked turkey and continue cooking for 3 minutes or until the sauce has evaporated. Top with cheddar and serve.

Buttery Broccoli and Bacon

Preparation Time: 5 minutes

Cooking Time: 10 minutes

Servings: 2

Ingredients:

- 1 slice of turkey bacon
- 1 cup chopped broccoli florets
- 1/8 teaspoon garlic powder
- ¼ teaspoon Italian seasoning
- ¼ tablespoon unsalted butter

EXTRA:

- 1/8 teaspoon salt
- 1/8 teaspoon ground black pepper

Directions:

1. Take a medium skillet pan, place it over high heat, add bacon slice and cook for 3 to 5 minutes until crispy.
2. Transfer bacon to a cutting board and then chop it into small pieces.
3. Reduce the heat to medium-low level, add broccoli florets into the pan, stir well into the bacon grease, add butter, then toss until mixed and cook for 5 minutes until tender.
4. Season the broccoli florets with salt, black pepper, and Italian seasoning, add chopped bacon, stir well and cook for 2 minutes until thoroughly heated.

Creamy Curry Noodles

Preparation Time: 19 minutes

Cooking Time: 10 minutes

Servings: 4

Ingredients:

CREAMY CURRY SAUCE

- Apple cider vinegar, two tablespoons
- Water, one-quarter of one cup
- Avocado oil, two tablespoons
- Turmeric, ground, one teaspoon
- Black pepper, one half teaspoon
- Tahini, one-quarter of one cup
- Coriander, ground, one- and one-half teaspoons
- Cumin, ground, one teaspoon
- Salt, one teaspoon
- Curry powder, two teaspoons
- Ginger, ground, one quarter teaspoon

NOODLE BOWL

- Cilantro, fresh, chopped small, one half cup
- Bell pepper, red, one cleaned and diced
- Zucchini noodles, one sixteen-ounce pack
- Carrots, two, peeled and cut in julienne strips
- Kale, two cups packed
- Cauliflower, one half of one head chopped small

Directions:

1. Cover the zucchini noodles with two cups of boiling water in a medium-sized bowl and set them off to the side. After leaving the noodles in the water for five minutes, drain off the water and place the noodles back into the bowl. Prep all of the veggies and then toss them into the bowl with the noodles. Toss the ingredients in the bowl gently, but well.
2. Divide the leaves of kale onto four serving plates. Mix the list of ingredients for the Creamy Curry Sauce and blend them until they are smooth and creamy. When the sauce is well mixed, then pour it over the ingredients in the bowl and toss the ingredients well until all are covered with the sauce.
3. Then divide the noodles over the kale on the four plates and serve.

Roasted Vegetables

Preparation Time: 10 minutes

Cooking Time: 20 minutes

Servings: 4

Ingredients:

- Cilantro, chopped, one-quarter of one cup
- Green onion, diced, one half of one cup

MASALA SEASONING

- Black pepper, one half teaspoon
- Turmeric, one quarter teaspoon
- Chili powder, ground, one half teaspoon
- Tomato puree, one half of one cup
- Garam masala, one quarter teaspoon

- Salt, one half teaspoon
- Garlic, minced, one tablespoon
- Olive oil, two tablespoons
- Ginger, ground, two teaspoons

VEGGIES

- Cauliflower, one cup in small pieces
- Mushrooms, sliced one half of one cup
- Green beans, three-fourths of one cup

Directions:

1. Heat the oven to 400. Place the rack in the oven in the middle. Use aluminum foil or parchment paper to cover a baking sheet completely. Chop the veggies if they are not already chopped. Use a medium-sized bowl to mix the chili powder, ginger, garam masala, garlic, pepper, salt, and the tomato puree, making sure the ingredients are all mixed well.
2. Then mix in the olive oil. Place the chopped veggies into this mixture and mix them in well. Then place the coated veggies onto the covered baking sheet in one single layer.
3. Roast the veggies in the heated oven for thirty to forty minutes or until the veggies are cooked in a manner in which you like them.

Green Pea Fritter

Preparation Time: 10 minutes
Cooking Time: 20 minutes
Servings: 4
Ingredients:

- Frozen peas, two cups
- Olive oil, one tablespoon + one tablespoon
- Onion, one diced
- Garlic, three tablespoons

- Chickpea flour, one- and one-half cups
- Baking soda, one teaspoon
- Salt, one quarter teaspoon
- Rosemary, one teaspoon
- Thyme, one half teaspoon
- Marjoram, one teaspoon
- Lemon juice, two tablespoons

Directions:

1. Heat the oven to 350°F. Use spray oil to spray a baking sheet. Boil the peas for five minutes.
2. Pour one tablespoon of olive oil in a skillet and fry the garlic and onion for five minutes.
3. Pour the garlic and onion with the olive oil in a bowl and add the cooked peas, mashing them until they make a thick paste. Blend in the marjoram, thyme, rosemary, salt, baking soda, and chickpea flour.
4. Dampen your hands and form the mash into ten equal-sized patties. Brush the patties with the other tablespoon of olive oil. Bake them for 18 minutes in the oven, turning them over after 9 minutes. Serve immediately!

Roasted Mushrooms and Shallots

Preparation Time: 10 minutes
Cooking Time: 20 minutes
Servings: 4
Ingredients:

- Mushrooms, fresh, one-pound cut into bite-size pieces

- Shallots, two cups sliced thick
- Olive oil, two tablespoons
- Thyme, dried, one teaspoon
- Salt, one quarter teaspoon
- Black pepper, one quarter teaspoon
- Red wine vinegar, one third cup

Directions:

1. Preheat your oven to 450°F.
2. Place the shallots and mushrooms in a large bowl and add salt, pepper, thyme, and olive oil and toss the ingredients together to coat the shallots and mushrooms thoroughly.
3. Roast the veggies on a baking sheet for fifteen minutes. Pour the red wine vinegar over the veggies and bake for five more minutes.

Garlic Chili Roasted Kohlrabi

Preparation Time: 5 minutes
Cooking Time: 12 minutes
Servings: 1
Ingredients:

- Olive oil, two tablespoons
- Garlic, minced, one tablespoon
- Chili pepper, one teaspoon
- Salt, one quarter teaspoon
- Kohlrabi, one and one-half pounds, peel and cut into one half inch wedges
- Cilantro, fresh, chopped, two tablespoons

Directions:

1. Heat your oven to 450°F. Mix in a large bowl, the pepper, salt, chili pepper, garlic, and olive oil. Put in the kohlrabi and toss well to coat the kohlrabi.
2. Bake the coated kohlrabi for twenty minutes, stirring it around when you are about halfway done with cooking. Sprinkle on the cilantro and serve.

Vegetarian Nachos

Preparation Time: 15 minutes
Cooking Time: 0 minutes
Servings: 6
Ingredients:

- Pita chips, whole wheat, three cups
- Nutritional yeast, one half cup
- Oregano, dried, one tablespoon minced
- Romaine lettuce, one cup chopped
- Grape tomatoes, one-half cup cut in quarters
- Olive oil, two tablespoons
- Lemon juice, one tablespoon
- Hummus, one-third cup prepared
- Black pepper, one half teaspoon
- Red onion, two tablespoons minced
- Tofu, one-half cup cut into small crumbles
- Black olives, two tablespoons chopped

Directions:

1. Mix the hummus, pepper, olive oil, and lemon juice in a mixing bowl. Spread a layer of the pita chips on a serving platter.
2. Drizzle three-fourths of the hummus mix over the pita chips. Use the lettuce, red onion, tomatoes, and olives to garnish the hummus.
3. Make a small mound of the leftover hummus in the middle of the chips, then garnish all with the oregano and the nutritional yeast.

VEGAN Macaroni and Cheese

Preparation Time: 15 minutes
Cooking Time: 20 minutes
Servings: 4
Ingredients:

- Elbow macaroni, whole grain, eight ounces, cooked
- Nutritional yeast, one quarter cup
- Garlic, minced, two tablespoons
- Apple cider vinegar, two teaspoons
- Broccoli, one head with florets cut into bite-sized pieces
- Water, one cup (more if needed)

- Garlic powder, one half teaspoon
- Avocado oil, two tablespoons
- Red pepper, flakes, one eighth teaspoon
- Onion, yellow, chopped, one cup
- Salt, one half teaspoon
- Russet potato, peeled and grated, one cup (about two small potatoes)
- Dry mustard powder, one half teaspoon
- Onion powder, one half teaspoon

Directions:

1. Cook the broccoli for five minutes in boiling water. Add the cooked broccoli to the cooked pasta in a large mixing bowl.
2. Cook the onion in the avocado oil for five minutes, then stir in the red pepper flakes, garlic, salt, mustard powder, garlic powder, grated potato, and onion powder. Cook this for three minutes and then pour in the water and mix well. Cook this for eight to ten minutes or until the potatoes are soft.
3. Pour all of this mixture carefully into a blender and add in the nutritional yeast and the vinegar and then blend. When this is creamy and smooth, then pour it into the mixing bowl and mix well with the broccoli and pasta.

Cilantro Lime Coleslaw

Preparation Time: 5 minutes

Cooking Time: 0 minutes

Servings: 5

Ingredients:

- Avocados, two
- Garlic, minced, one tablespoon
- Coleslaw, ready-made in a bag, fourteen ounces
- Cilantro, fresh leaves, one-quarter cup minced
- Salt, one half teaspoon
- Lime juice, two tablespoons
- Water, one quarter cup

Directions:

1. Except for the slaw mix, put all of the ingredients that are listed into a blender. Blend these ingredients well until they are creamy and smooth.
2. Mix the coleslaw mix in with this dressing and then toss it gently to mix it well.
3. Keep the mixed coleslaw in the refrigerator until you are ready to serve.

Delicious Broccoli

Preparation Time: 15 minutes

Cooking Time: 15 minutes

Servings: 8

Ingredients:

- 2 oranges, sliced in half
- 1 lb. broccoli rabe
- 2 tablespoons sesame oil, toasted
- Salt and pepper to taste
- 1 tablespoon sesame seeds, toasted

Directions:

1. Pour the oil into a pan over medium heat.
2. Add the oranges and cook until caramelized and transfer to a plate.
3. Put the broccoli in the pan and cook for 8 minutes.
4. Squeeze the oranges to release juice in a bowl, add oil, salt, and pepper and coat the broccoli rabe with the mixture. Sprinkle seeds on top.

Spicy Peanut Soba Noodles

Preparation Time: 7 minutes

Cooking Time: 17 minutes

Servings: 1

Ingredients:

- 5 ounces uncooked soba noodles
- ½ tablespoon low sodium soy sauce
- 1 clove garlic, minced

- 4 teaspoons water
- 1 small head broccoli, cut into florets
- ½ cup carrot
- ¼ cup finely chopped scallions
- 3 tablespoons peanut butter
- 1 tablespoon honey
- 1 teaspoon crushed red pepper flakes
- 2 teaspoons vegetable oil
- 4 ounces button mushrooms, discard stems
- 3 tablespoons peanuts, dry roasted, unsalted

Directions:

1. Cook soba noodles following the directions on the package.
2. Add peanut butter, honey, water, soy sauce, garlic, and red pepper flakes. Whisk until well combined.
3. Place a skillet over medium heat. Add oil. When the oil is heated, add broccoli and sauté for a few minutes until crisp as well as tender. Add mushrooms and sauté until the mushrooms are tender. Turn off the heat.
4. Add the sauce mixture and carrots and mix well.
5. Crush the peanuts by rolling with a rolling pin.
6. Divide the noodles into bowls. Pour sauce mixture over it. Sprinkle scallions and peanuts on top and serve.

Dinner Recipes

Garlic Zucchini and Cauliflower

Preparation Time: 10 minutes
Cooking Time: 20 minutes
Servings: 4
Ingredients:

- 4 zucchinis, cut into medium fries
- 1 cup cauliflower florets
- 1 tablespoon capers, drained
- Juice of ½ lemon
- A pinch of salt and black pepper
- ½ teaspoon chili powder
- 1 tablespoon olive oil
- ¼ teaspoon garlic powder

Directions:

1. Spread the zucchini fries on a lined baking sheet, add the rest of the ingredients, toss, introduce in the oven, bake at 400 degrees F for 20 minutes, divide between plates and serve.

Garlic Beans

Preparation Time: 10 minutes
Cooking Time: 10 minutes
Servings: 4
Ingredients:

- Juice of 1 lemon
- Zest of 1 lemon, grated
- 2 tablespoons avocado oil
- 4 garlic cloves, minced
- ½ teaspoon turmeric powder
- 1 teaspoon garam masala
- 1 red onion, sliced
- 1 yellow bell pepper, sliced
- 10 ounces green beans, halved
- A pinch of black pepper

Directions:

1. Heat up a pan with the oil over medium-high heat, add the garlic and onion and cook for 2 minutes.
2. Add green beans and the other ingredients, toss, cook for 8 minutes, divide between plates and serve.

Mustard Beets

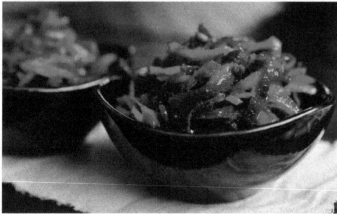

Preparation Time: 10 minutes
Cooking Time: 0 minutes
Servings: 4
Ingredients:

- 1 tablespoon Dijon mustard
- 1 and ½ tablespoon olive oil
- 8 ounces beets, cooked and sliced
- 1 teaspoon garam masala
- 1 teaspoon coriander, ground
- 1 teaspoon basil, dried
- A pinch of black pepper

Directions:

1. In a bowl, mix the beets with the oil, mustard and the other ingredients, toss and serve.

Parsley Green Beans

Preparation Time: 10 minutes
Cooking Time: 20 minutes
Servings: 6

Ingredients:

- 3 tablespoons olive oil

36

- 3 pounds green beans, halved
- A pinch of salt and black pepper
- 2 tablespoons balsamic vinegar
- 2 yellow onions, chopped
- 2 and ½ tablespoons parsley, chopped

Directions:
1. Heat a pan with the oil over medium heat, add the green beans and the other ingredients, toss, cook for 20 minutes, divide between plates and serve.

Squash and Tomatoes

Preparation Time: 15 minutes
Cooking Time: 12 minutes
Servings: 2
Ingredients:
- 8 oz yellow squash, peeled and roughly cubed
- 1 cup cherry tomatoes, halved
- 3 tablespoons tomato sauce
- 1 teaspoon sweet paprika
- 1 teaspoon coriander, ground
- 1 teaspoon oregano, dried
- 1 teaspoon olive oil
- 1 teaspoon white pepper

Directions:
1. Heat up a pan with the oil over medium heat, add the squash, tomatoes and the other ingredients.
2. Cook for 12 minutes on low heat.
3. Transfer into plates and serve.

Bok Choy Salad

Preparation Time: 10 minutes
Cooking Time: 10 minutes
Servings: 5
Ingredients:
- 10 oz bok choy, chopped
- 1 cup cherry tomatoes, halved
- 1 tablespoon black olives, pitted and sliced
- 1 mango, peeled and cubed
- Juice of ½ orange
- 1 teaspoon curry powder
- 1 teaspoon sesame oil
- 1 tablespoon lemon juice

Directions:
1. Heat up a pan with the oil over medium-high heat, add the bok choy, tomatoes and the other ingredients, toss and cook for 10 minutes.
2. Divide into bowls and serve cold.

Balsamic Arugula and Beets

Preparation Time: 10 minutes
Cooking Time: 0 minutes
Servings: 4
Ingredients:
- 2 cups baby arugula
- 1 tablespoon balsamic vinegar
- 1 teaspoon olive oil
- 2 red beets, baked, peeled and cubed
- 1 avocado, peeled, pitted and cubed
- 1 teaspoon marsala
- ½ teaspoon salt
- ½ teaspoon cayenne pepper

Directions:
1. In a bowl, mix the arugula with the beets and the vinegar. Mix and add olive oil, chopped avocado and marsala, salt and pepper. Mix well.
2. Serve and enjoy.

Herbed Beets

Preparation Time: 10 minutes
Cooking Time: 40 minutes
Servings: 3
Ingredients:

- 2 big red beets, peeled and roughly cubed
- 1 tablespoon chives, chopped
- 1 tablespoon cilantro, chopped
- 1 tablespoon basil, chopped
- Juice of 1 lime
- A pinch of salt and black pepper
- ¼ teaspoon dried oregano
- ¼ teaspoon ground nutmeg
- ¼ teaspoon ground cumin
- 1 tablespoon olive oil

Directions:

1. Preheat oven to 400°F. Take a baking dish with parchment paper.
2. Take a bowl and place in the chives, cilantro and beets. Add basil, salt, pepper and lime juice and mix well. Add sprinkle the oregano, nutmeg, and cumin. Pour a tablespoon of olive oil and mix well.
3. Transfer in the baking dish and bake for 40 minutes.
4. Divide between plates and serve.

Marinara Broccoli

Preparation Time: 10 minutes
Cooking Time: 15 minutes
Servings: 4
Ingredients:

- 2 cups broccoli florets
- 1 teaspoon sweet paprika
- 1 teaspoon coriander, ground
- ¼ cup marinara sauce
- ½ teaspoon ground black pepper
- ½ teaspoon salt
- ½ teaspoon garlic powder
- 1 teaspoon olive oil
- Juice of 1 lime

Directions:

1. In a roasting pan, mix the broccoli with the marinara and the other ingredients, toss and bake at 400 degrees F for 15 minutes.
2. Divide between plates and serve.

Spinach and Pear Salad

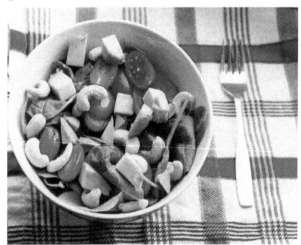

Preparation Time: 10 minutes
Cooking Time: 0 minutes
Servings: 2
Ingredients:

- 1 bell pepper, chopped
- ½ cup radishes, halved
- ½ cup cherry tomatoes, halved
- 2 cups baby spinach
- 2 pears, cored and cut into wedges
- 1 tablespoon walnuts, chopped
- 1 teaspoon chives, chopped
- A pinch of salt and black pepper
- Juice of 1 lime

Directions:

1. In a bowl, mix the radishes with the pepper, tomatoes and the other ingredients.

2. Serve and enjoy.

Olives and Mango Mix
Preparation Time: 10 minutes
Cooking Time: 0 minutes
Servings: 2
Ingredients:
- 1 cup black olives, pitted and halved
- 1 cup kalamata olives, pitted and halved

- 1 cup mango, peeled and cubed
- A pinch of salt and black pepper
- Juice of 1 lime
- 1 teaspoon sweet paprika
- 1 teaspoon coriander, ground
- 1 tablespoon olive oil

Directions:
1. In a bowl mix the olives with the mango and the other ingredients, toss and serve.

Eggplant and Avocado Mix
Preparation Time: 10 minutes
Cooking Time: 20 minutes
Servings: 4
Ingredients:
- 1-pound eggplant, roughly cubed
- 2 avocados, peeled, pitted and cubed
- 1 red onion, chopped

- 1 teaspoon curry powder
- Juice of 1 lime
- ½ cup crushed tomatoes
- 1 tablespoon olive oil
- 1 teaspoon salt
- 1 teaspoon chili powder

Directions:
1. Heat up a pan with the oil over medium heat, add the onion and cook for 5 minutes.
2. Add the eggplants, avocados and the other ingredients, toss and cook for 15 minutes more.
3. Divide between plates and serve.

Red Onion, Avocado and Radishes Mix
Preparation Time: 15 minutes
Cooking Time: 12 minutes
Servings: 2
Ingredients:
- 2 red onions, peeled and sliced
- 2 avocados, peeled, pitted and sliced

- 1 cup radishes, halved
- 1 teaspoon oregano, dried
- 1 teaspoon basil, dried
- 1 tablespoon olive oil
- 1 teaspoon lemon juice
- ¼ teaspoon salt

Directions:
1. Heat a pan with the oil over medium heat, add the onions, oregano and basil and cook for 5 minutes.
2. Add the rest of the ingredients, toss, cook for 7 minutes more, divide into bowls and serve.

Cajun and Balsamic Okra
Preparation Time: 10 minutes
Cooking Time: 15 minutes
Servings: 2
Ingredients:
- 1 cup okra, sliced
- ½ cup crushed tomatoes
- 1 teaspoon Cajun seasoning

- 2 tablespoons balsamic vinegar
- 1 teaspoon salt
- 1 teaspoon ground black pepper

- 1 tablespoon fresh parsley, chopped
- 1 teaspoon olive oil

Directions:
1. Heat up a pan with the oil over medium heat, add the okra, seasoning and the remaining ingredients, toss and cook for 15 minutes.
2. Divide into bowls and serve.

Cashew Zucchinis

Preparation Time: 10 minutes
Cooking Time: 40 minutes
Servings: 4
Ingredients:
- 1-pound zucchinis, sliced
- ½ cup cashews, soaked for a couple of hours and drained
- 1 cup coconut milk
- ¼ teaspoon nutmeg, ground
- 1 teaspoon chili powder
- A pinch of salt and black pepper

Directions:
1. In a roasting pan, mix the zucchinis with the cashews and the other ingredients, toss gently and cook at 380 degrees F for 40 minutes.
2. Divide into bowls and serve.

BOOK 2: DELICIOUS RECIPES

AND 21-DAY MEAL PLAN

Soup and Stew Recipes

Winter Comfort Stew

Preparation Time: 15 minutes

Cooking Time: 50 minutes

Servings: 6

Ingredients:

- 2 tbsp. olive oil
- 1 small yellow onion, chopped
- 2 garlic cloves, chopped
- 2 lb. grass-fed beef chuck, cut into 1-inch cubes
- 1 (14-oz.) can sugar-free crushed tomatoes
- 2 tsp. ground allspice
- 1½ tsp. red pepper flakes
- ½ C. homemade beef broth
- 6 oz. green olives, pitted
- 8 oz. fresh baby spinach
- 2 tbsp. fresh lemon juice
- Salt and freshly ground black pepper, to taste
- ¼ C. fresh cilantro, chopped

Directions:

1. In a pan, heat the oil over high heat and sauté the onion and garlic for about 2-3 minutes.
2. Add the beef and cook for about 3-4 minutes or until browned, stirring frequently.
3. Add the tomatoes, spices and broth and bring to a boil.
4. Reduce the heat to low and simmer, covered for about 30-40 minutes or until the beef's desired doneness.
5. Stir in the olives and spinach and simmer for about 2-3 minutes.
6. Stir in the lemon juice, salt and black pepper and remove from the heat.
7. Serve hot with the garnishing of cilantro.

Ideal Cold Weather Stew

Preparation Time: 20 minutes

Cooking Time: 2 hours 40 minutes

Servings: 6

Ingredients:

- 3 tbsp. olive oil, divided
- 8 oz. fresh mushrooms, quartered
- 1¼ lb. grass-fed beef chuck roast, trimmed and cubed into 1-inch size
- 2 tbsp. tomato paste
- ½ tsp. dried thyme
- 1 bay leaf
- 5 C. homemade beef broth
- 6 oz. celery root, peeled and cubed
- 4 oz. yellow onions, chopped roughly
- 3 oz. carrot, peeled and sliced
- 2 garlic cloves, sliced
- Salt and freshly ground black pepper, to taste

Directions:

1. In a Dutch oven, heat 1 tbsp. of the oil over medium heat and cook the mushrooms for about 2 minutes, without stirring.
2. Stir the mushroom and cook for about 2 minutes more.
3. With a slotted spoon, transfer the mushroom onto a plate.
4. In the same pan, heat the remaining oil over medium-high heat and sear the beef cubes for about 4-5 minutes.
5. Stir in the tomato paste, thyme and bay leaf and cook for about 1 minute.
6. Stir in the broth and bring to a boil.
7. Reduce the heat to low and simmer, covered for about 1½ hours.
8. Stir in the mushrooms, celery, onion, carrot and garlic and simmers for about 40-60 minutes.
9. Stir in the salt and black pepper and remove from the heat.
10. Serve hot.

Weekend Dinner Stew

Preparation Time: 15 minutes
Cooking Time: 55 minutes
Servings: 6
Ingredients:

- 1½ lb. grass-fed beef stew meat, trimmed and cubed into 1-inch size
- Salt and freshly ground black pepper, to taste
- 1 tbsp. olive oil
- 1 C. homemade tomato puree
- 4 C. homemade beef broth
- 2 C. zucchini, chopped
- 2 celery ribs, sliced
- ½ C. carrots, peeled and sliced
- 2 garlic cloves, minced
- ½ tbsp. dried thyme
- 1 tsp. dried parsley
- 1 tsp. dried rosemary
- 1 tbsp. paprika
- 1 tsp. onion powder
- 1 tsp. garlic powder

Directions:

1. In a large bowl, add the beef cubes, salt and black pepper and toss to coat well.
2. In a large pan, heat the oil over medium-high heat and cook the beef cubes for about 4-5 minutes or until browned.
3. Add the remaining ingredients and stir to combine.
4. Increase the heat to high and bring to a boil.
5. Reduce the heat to low and simmer, covered for about 40-50 minutes.
6. Stir in the salt and black pepper and remove from the heat. Serve hot.

Mexican Pork Stew

Preparation Time: 15 minutes
Cooking Time: 2 hours 10 minutes
Servings: 1
Ingredients:

- 3 tbsp. unsalted butter
- 2½ lb. boneless pork ribs, cut into ¾-inch cubes
- 1 large yellow onion, chopped
- 4 garlic cloves, crushed
- 1½ C. homemade chicken broth
- 2 (10-oz.) cans sugar-free diced tomatoes
- 1 C. canned roasted poblano chiles
- 2 tsp. dried oregano
- 1 tsp. ground cumin
- Salt, to taste
- ¼ C. fresh cilantro, chopped
- 2 tbsp. fresh lime juice

Directions:

1. In a large pan, melt the butter over medium-high heat and cook the pork, onions and garlic for about 5 minutes or until browned. Add the broth and scrape up the browned bits.
2. Add the tomatoes, poblano chiles, oregano, cumin, and salt and bring to a boil.
3. Reduce the heat to medium-low and simmer, covered for about 2 hours.
4. Stir in the fresh cilantro and lime juice and remove from heat. Serve hot.

Hungarian Pork Stew

Preparation Time: 15 minutes
Cooking Time: 2 hours 20 minutes
Servings: 10
Ingredients:

- 3 tbsp. olive oil
- 3½ lb. pork shoulder, cut into 4 portions
- 1 tbsp. butter
- 2 medium onions, chopped
- 16 oz. tomatoes, crushed
- 5 garlic cloves, crushed

- 2 Hungarian wax peppers, chopped
- 3 tbsp. Hungarian Sweet paprika
- 1 tbsp. smoked paprika
- 1 tsp. hot paprika
- ½ tsp. caraway seeds
- 1 bay leaf

- 1 C. homemade chicken broth
- 1 packet unflavored gelatin
- 2 tbsp. fresh lemon juice
- Pinch of xanthan gum
- Salt and freshly ground black pepper, to taste

Directions:

1. In a heavy-bottomed pan, heat 1 tbsp. of oil over high heat and sear the pork for about 2-3 minutes or until browned. Transfer the pork onto a plate and cut into bite-sized pieces.
2. In the same pan, heat 1 tbsp. of oil and butter over medium-low heat and sauté the onions for about 5-6 minutes.
3. With a slotted spoon transfer the onion into a bowl.
4. In the same pan, add the tomatoes and cook for about 3-4 minutes, without stirring.
5. Meanwhile, in a small frying pan, heat the remaining oil over-low heat and sauté the garlic, wax peppers, all kinds of paprika and caraway seeds for about 20-30 seconds.
6. Remove from the heat and set aside.
7. In a small bowl, mix together the gelatin and broth.
8. In the large pan, add the cooked pork, garlic mixture, gelatin mixture and bay leaf and bring to a gentle boil.
9. Reduce the heat to low and simmer, covered for about 2 hours.
10. Stir in the xanthan gum and simmer for about 3-5 minutes.
11. Stir in the lemon juice, salt and black pepper and remove from the heat. Serve hot.

Yellow Chicken Soup

Preparation Time: 15 minutes
Cooking Time: 25 minutes
Servings: 5
Ingredients:

- 2½ tsp. ground turmeric
- 1½ tsp. ground cumin
- 1/8 tsp cayenne pepper
- 2 tbsp. butter, divided
- 1 small yellow onion, chopped
- 2 C. cauliflower, chopped

- 2 C. broccoli, chopped
- 4 C. homemade chicken broth
- 1½ C. water
- 1 tsp. fresh ginger root, grated
- 1 bay leaf
- 2 C. Swiss chard, stemmed and chopped finely
- ½ C. unsweetened coconut milk
- 3 (4-oz.) grass-fed boneless, skinless chicken thighs, cut into bite-size pieces
- 2 tbsp. fresh lime juice

Directions:

1. In a small bowl, mix together the turmeric, cumin and cayenne pepper and set aside.
2. In a large pan, melt 1 tbsp. of the butter over medium heat and sauté the onion for about 3-4 minutes.
3. Add the cauliflower, broccoli and half of the spice mixture and cook for another 3-4 minutes.
4. Add the broth, water, ginger and bay leaf and bring to a boil.
5. Reduce the heat to low and simmer for about 8-10 minutes.
6. Stir in the Swiss chard and coconut milk and cook for about 1-2 minutes.
7. Meanwhile, in a large skillet, melt the remaining butter over medium heat and sear the chicken pieces for about 5 minutes. Stir in the remaining spice mix and cook for about 5 minutes, stirring frequently.
8. Transfer the soup into serving bowls and top with the chicken pieces. Drizzle with lime juice and serve.

Curry Soup

Preparation Time: 25 minutes
Cooking Time: 20 minutes
Servings: 4
Ingredients:

- ¾ tsp. cumin
- ¼ c. pumpkin seeds, raw
- ½ tsp. garlic powder
- ½ tsp. paprika ½ tsp. sea salt
- 1 c. coconut milk, unsweetened
- 1 clove garlic, minced
- 1 med. onion, diced
- 2 carrots, chopped
- 2 tbsp. curry powder
- 3 c. cauliflower, riced
- 3 tbsp. extra virgin olive oil, divided
- 4 c. kale, chopped
- 4 c. vegetable broth
- Sea salt and pepper, to taste

Directions:

1. Hear a large sauté pan over medium heat with 2 tablespoons of olive oil. Once the oil is hot, add the rice cauliflower to the pan and the curry powder, cumin, salt, paprika, and garlic powder. Stir thoroughly to combine.
2. While cooking, stir occasionally. Once the cauliflower is warmed through, remove it from the heat.
3. In a large pot over medium heat, add the remainder of your olive oil. Once it's hot, add the onion and allow it to cook for about four minutes. Add the garlic, then cook for about another two minutes.
4. To the large pot, add the broth, kale, carrots, and cauliflower. Stir to incorporate thoroughly.
5. Allow the mixture to come to a boil, drop the heat to low, and allow the soup to simmer for about 15 minutes.
6. Stir the coconut milk into the mixture along with salt and pepper to taste.
7. Garnish with pumpkin seeds and serve hot!

Delicious Tomato Basil Soup

Preparation Time: 10 minutes
Cook Time: 40 minutes
Servings: 4
Ingredients:

- ¼ c. olive oil
- ½ c. heavy cream
- 1 lb. tomatoes, fresh
- 4 c. chicken broth, divided
- 4 cloves garlic, fresh
- Sea salt and pepper, to taste

Directions:

1. Preheat oven to 400° Fahrenheit and line a baking sheet with foil.
2. Remove the cores from your tomatoes and place them on the baking sheet along with the cloves of garlic.
3. Drizzle tomatoes and garlic with olive oil, salt, and pepper.
4. Roast at 400° Fahrenheit for 30 minutes.
5. Pull the tomatoes out of the oven and place into a blender, along with the juices that have dripped onto the pan during roasting. Add two cups of the chicken broth to the blender.
6. Blend until smooth, then strain the mixture into a large saucepan or a pot.
7. While the pan is on the stove, whisk the remaining two cups of broth and the cream into the soup.
8. Simmer for about ten minutes. Season to taste, then serve hot!

Chicken Enchilada Soup

Preparation Time: 10 minutes
Cooking Time: 45 minutes
Servings: 4
Ingredients:

- ½ c. fresh cilantro, chopped

- 1 ¼ tsp. chili powder
- 1 c. fresh tomatoes, diced
- 1 med. yellow onion, diced
- 1 sm. red bell pepper, diced
- 1 tbsp. cumin, ground
- 1 tbsp. extra virgin olive oil
- 1 tbsp. lime juice, fresh
- 1 tsp. dried oregano
- 2 cloves garlic, minced
- 2 lg. stalks celery, diced
- 4 c. chicken broth
- 8 oz. chicken thighs, boneless and skinless, shredded
- 8 oz. cream cheese, softened

Directions:
1. In a pot over medium heat, warm olive oil.
2. Once hot, add celery, red pepper, onion, and garlic. Cook for about 3 minutes or until shiny.
3. Stir the tomatoes into the pot and let cook for another 2 minutes.
4. Add seasonings to the pot, stir in chicken broth and bring to a boil.
5. Once boiling, drop the heat down to low and allow to simmer for 20 minutes.
6. Once simmered, add the cream cheese and allow the soup to return to a boil.
7. Drop the heat once again and allow to simmer for another 20 minutes. Stir the shredded chicken into the soup along with the lime juice and the cilantro. Spoon into bowls and serve hot!

Buffalo Chicken Soup
Preparation Time: 20 minutes
Cook Time: 20 minutes
Servings: 4
Ingredients:
- 4 med. stalks celery, diced
- 2 med. carrots, diced
- 4 chicken breasts, boneless and skinless
- 6 tbsp. butter
- 1 qt. chicken broth
- 2 oz. cream cheese
- ½ c. heavy cream
- ½ c. buffalo sauce 1 tsp. sea salt
- ½ tsp. thyme, dried

FOR GARNISH
- Sour cream
- Green onions, thinly sliced
- Bleu cheese crumbles

Directions:
1. Set a large pot to warm over medium heat with the olive oil in it.
2. Cook celery and carrot until shiny and tender. Add chicken breasts to the pot and cover. Allow to cook about five to six minutes per side. Once the chicken has cooked and formed some caramelization on each side, remove it from the pot.
3. Shred the chicken breasts and set aside. Pour the chicken broth into the pot with the carrots and celery, then stir in the cream, butter, and cream cheese. * Bring the pot to a boil, then add chicken back to the pot. Stir buffalo sauce into the mix and combine completely. Feel free to increase or decrease as desired.
4. Add seasonings, stir, and drop the heat to low. Allow the soup to simmer for 15 to 20 minutes, or until all the flavors have fully combined. Serve hot with a garnish of sour cream, bleu cheese crumbles, and sliced green onion!

Slow Cooker Taco Soup
Preparation Time: 10 minutes
Cooking Time: 2 hours
Servings: 8
Ingredients:
- ¼ c. sour cream

- ½ c. cheddar cheese, shredded
- 2 c. diced tomatoes
- 2 lbs. ground beef
- 3 tbsp. taco seasoning
- 4 c. chicken broth
- 8 oz. cream cheese, cubed

Directions:

1. Heat a medium saucepan over medium heat and brown the beef. Drain the fat from the beef and then place it into the slow cooker. Add the cream cheese cubes, taco seasoning, and diced tomatoes into the slow cooker.
2. Add the chicken broth, cover and leave to cook on high for two hours.
3. Once the timer is up, stir all the ingredients and spoon the soup into bowls.
4. Serve hot with sour cream and shredded cheese on top!

Wedding Soup

Preparation Time: 5 minutes
Cooking Time: 10 minutes
Servings: 4
Ingredients:

- ½ c. almond flour
- ½ c. parmesan cheese, grated
- ½ sm. yellow onion, diced
- 1 lb. ground beef
- 1 lg. egg, beaten
- 1 tsp. Italian seasoning
- 1 tsp. oregano, fresh & chopped
- 1 tsp. thyme, fresh & chopped
- 2 c. baby leaf spinach, fresh
- 2 c. cauliflower, riced
- 2 med. stalks celery, diced
- 2 tbsp. extra virgin olive oil
- 3 cloves garlic, minced
- 6 c. chicken broth
- Sea salt and pepper, to taste

Directions:

1. In a large mixing bowl, combine almond flour, parmesan cheese, ground beef, egg, salt, pepper, and Italian seasoning. Mix thoroughly by band.
2. Shape the meat mixture into one-inch meatballs, cover, and refrigerate until ready to cook.
3. In a large saucepan over medium heat, warm the olive oil.
4. Once the oil is hot, stir the celery and onion into the pan and season to taste with salt and pepper.
5. Stirring often, bring the onion and celery to a lightly cooked state, about six or seven minutes.
6. Add the garlic to the pan, stir to combine, and allow to cook for one minute.
7. Stir chicken broth, fresh oregano, and the fresh thyme into the pan and stir to combine.
8. Bring the mixture to a boil. Drop the heat to low and simmer for about ten minutes before adding cauliflower and meatballs. Allow to cook for about five minutes or until the meatballs are cooked all the way through.
9. Add the spinach to the soup and stir in for about one to two minutes, or until it's sufficiently wilted.
10. Add seasoning as is needed. Serve hot!

Sweet Potato, Corn and Jalapeno Bisque

Preparation Time: 10 minutes
Cooking Time: 15 minutes
Servings: 4
Ingredients:

- 4 ears corn
- 1 seeded and chopped jalapeno
- 4 cups vegetable broth
- 1 tablespoon olive oil
- 3 peeled and cubed sweet potatoes
- 1 chopped onion
- ½ tablespoon salt
- ¼ teaspoon black pepper
- 1 minced garlic clove

Directions:

1. In a pan, heat the oil over medium flame and sauté onion and garlic in it and cook for around 3 minutes. Put broth and sweet potatoes in it and bring it to boil. Reduce the flame and cook it for an additional 10 minutes.
2. Remove it from the stove and blend it with a blender. Again, put it on the stove and add corn, jalapeno, salt, and black pepper and serve it.

Creamy Pea Soup with Olive Pesto

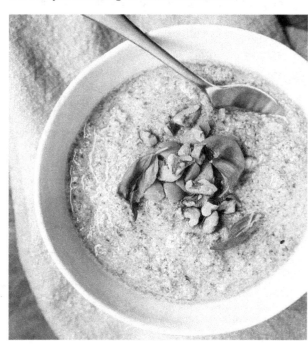

Preparation Time: 20 minutes
Cooking Time: 20 minutes
Servings: 4
Ingredients:

*   1 grated carrot
*   1 rinsed chopped leek
*   1 minced garlic clove
*   2 tablespoons olive oil
*   1 stem fresh thyme leaves
*   15 ounces rinsed and drained peas
*   ½ tablespoon salt
*   ¼ teaspoon ground black pepper
*   2 ½ cups vegetable broth
*   ¼ cup parsley leaves
*   1 ¼ cups pitted green olives
*   1 teaspoon drained capers
*   1 garlic clove

Directions:
1. Take a pan with oil and put it over medium flame and whisk garlic, leek, thyme, and carrot in it. Cook it for around 4 minutes. Add broth, peas, salt, and pepper and increase the heat. When it starts boiling, lower down the heat and cook it with a lid on for around 15 minutes and remove from heat and blend it.
2. For making pesto whisk parsley, olives, capers, and garlic and blend it, it has little chunks. Top the soup with the scoop of olive pesto.

Spinach Soup with Dill and Basil

Preparation Time: 10 minutes
Cooking Time: 25 minutes
Servings: 8
Ingredients:

*   1 pound peeled and diced potatoes
*   1 tablespoon minced garlic
*   1 teaspoon dry mustard
*   6 cups vegetable broth
*   20 ounces chopped frozen spinach
*   2 cups chopped onion
*   1 ½ tablespoons salt
*   ½ cup minced dill
*   1 cup basil
*   ½ teaspoon ground black pepper

Directions:
1. Whisk onion, garlic, potatoes, broth, mustard, and salt in a pan and cook it over medium flame. When it starts boiling, low down the heat and cover it with the lid and cook for 20 minutes.
2. Add the remaining ingredients in it and blend it and cook it for few more minutes and serve it.

Coconut Watercress Soup

Preparation Time: 10 minutes
Cooking Time: 20 minutes
Servings: 4
Ingredients:

- 1 teaspoon coconut oil
- 1 onion, diced
- ¾ cup coconut milk

Directions:

1. Melt the coconut oil in a large pot over medium-high heat. Add the onion and cook until soft, about 5 minutes, then add the peas and the water. Bring to a boil, lower the heat and add the watercress, mint, salt, and pepper.
2. Cover and simmer for 5 minutes. Stir in the coconut milk, and purée the soup until smooth in a blender or an immersion blender.
3. Try this soup with any other fresh, leafy green—anything from spinach to collard greens to arugula to swiss chard.

Roasted Red Pepper and Butternut Squash Soup

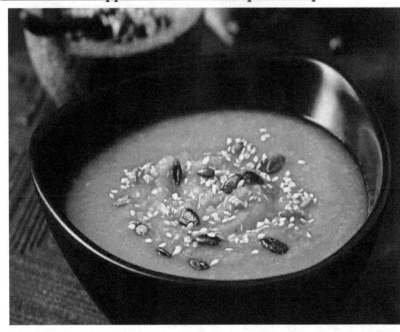

Preparation Time: 10 minutes
Cooking Time: 45 minutes
Servings: 6
Ingredients:

- 1 small butternut squash
- 1 tablespoon olive oil
- 1 teaspoon sea salt
- 2 red bell peppers
- 1 yellow onion
- 1 head garlic
- 2 cups water, or vegetable broth
- Zest and juice of 1 lime
- 1 to 2 tablespoons tahini
- Pinch cayenne pepper
- ½ teaspoon ground coriander
- ½ teaspoon ground cumin
- Toasted squash seeds (optional)

Directions:

1. Preheat the oven to 350°f.
2. Prepare the squash for roasting by cutting it in half lengthwise, scooping out the seeds, and poking holes in the flesh with a fork. Reserve the seeds if desired.
3. Rub a small amount of oil over the flesh and skin, rub with a bit of sea salt and put the halves skin-side down in a large baking dish. Put it in the oven while you prepare the rest of the vegetables.
4. Prepare the peppers the exact same way, except they do not need to be poked.
5. Slice the onion in half and rub oil on the exposed faces. Slice the top off the head of garlic and rub oil on the exposed flesh. After the squash has cooked for 20 minutes, add the peppers, onion, and garlic, and roast for another 20 minutes. Optionally, you can toast the squash seeds by putting them in the oven in a separate baking dish 10 to 15 minutes before the vegetables are finished.

6. Keep a close eye on them. When the vegetables are cooked, take them out and let them cool before handling them. The squash will be very soft when poked with a fork.
7. Scoop the flesh out of the squash skin into a large pot (if you have an immersion blender) or into a blender.
8. Chop the pepper roughly, remove the onion skin and chop the onion roughly, and squeeze the garlic cloves out of the head, all into the pot or blender. Add the water, the lime zest and juice, and the tahini. Purée the soup, adding more water if you like, to your desired consistency. Season with the salt, cayenne, coriander, and cumin. Serve garnished with toasted squash seeds.

Cauliflower Spinach Soup

Preparation Time: 30 minutes
Cooking Time: 25 minutes
Servings: 5
Ingredients:
- 1/2 cup unsweetened coconut milk
- 5 oz fresh spinach, chopped
- 5 watercress, chopped
- 8 cups vegetable stock
- 1 lb cauliflower, chopped
- Salt to taste

Directions:
1. Add stock and cauliflower in a large saucepan and bring to boil over medium heat for 15 minutes.
2. Add spinach and watercress and cook for another 10 minutes.
3. Remove from heat and puree the soup using a blender until smooth.
4. Add coconut milk and stir well. Season with salt. Stir well and serve hot.

Avocado Mint Soup

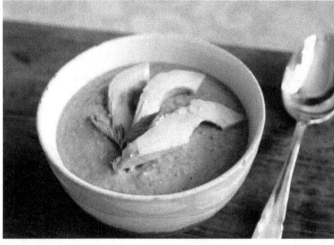

Preparation Time: 10 minutes
Cooking Time: 10 minutes
Servings: 2
Ingredients:
- 1 medium avocado, peeled, pitted, and cut into pieces
- 1 cup coconut milk
- 2 romaine lettuce leaves
- 20 fresh mint leaves
- 1 tbsp fresh lime juice
- 1/8 tsp salt

Directions:
1. Add all ingredients into the blender and blend until smooth. Soup should be thick not as a puree.
2. Pour into the serving bowls and place in the refrigerator for 10 minutes.
3. Stir well and serve chilled.

Creamy Squash Soup

Preparation Time: 10 minutes
Servings: 8

Servings: 8
Ingredients:
- 3 cups butternut squash, chopped
- 1 ½ cups unsweetened coconut milk
- 1 tbsp coconut oil
- 1 tsp dried onion flakes

- 1 tbsp curry powder
- 4 cups water
- 1 garlic clove
- 1 tsp kosher salt

Directions:

1. Add squash, coconut oil, onion flakes, curry powder, water, garlic, and salt into a large saucepan. Bring to boil over high heat.
2. Turn heat to medium and simmer for 20 minutes.
3. Puree the soup using a blender until smooth. Return soup to the saucepan and stir in coconut milk and cook for 2 minutes. Stir well and serve hot.

Zucchini Soup

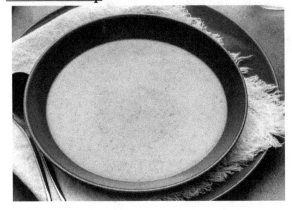

Preparation Time: 10 minutes

Cooking Time: 15 minutes

Servings: 8

Ingredients:

- 2 ½ lbs zucchini, peeled and sliced
- 1/3 cup basil leaves
- 4 cups vegetable stock
- 4 garlic cloves, chopped
- 2 tbsp olive oil
- 1 medium onion, diced
- Salt and pepper to taste

Directions:

1. Heat olive oil in a pan over medium-low heat.
2. Add zucchini and onion and sauté until softened. Add garlic and sauté for a minute.
3. Add vegetable stock and simmer for 15 minutes.
4. Remove from heat. Stir in basil and puree the soup using a blender until smooth and creamy. Season with pepper and salt. Stir well and serve.

Creamy Celery Soup

Preparation Time: 20 minutes

Cooking Time: 20 minutes

Servings: 4

Ingredients:

- 6 cups celery
- ½ tsp dill
- 2 cups water
- 1 cup coconut milk
- 1 onion, chopped
- Pinch of salt

Directions:

1. Add all ingredients into the electric pot and stir well.
2. Cover electric pot with the lid and select soup setting.
3. Release pressure using a quick release method than open the lid.
4. Puree the soup using an immersion blender until smooth and creamy.
5. Stir well and serve warm.

Avocado Cucumber Soup

Preparation Time: 20 minutes

Cooking Time: 0 minutes

Servings: 3

Ingredients:

- 1 large cucumber, peeled and sliced
- ¾ cup water
- ¼ cup lemon juice
- 2 garlic cloves
- 6 green onion
- 2 avocados, pitted
- ½ tsp black pepper
- ½ tsp pink salt

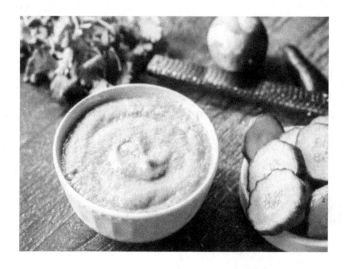

Directions:

1. Add all ingredients into the blender and blend until smooth and creamy.
2. Place in refrigerator for 30 minutes.
3. Stir well and serve chilled.

Garden Vegetable Stew

Preparation Time: 5 minutes

Cooking Time: 60 minutes

Servings: 4

Ingredients:

- 2 tablespoons olive oil
- 1 medium red onion, chopped
- 1 medium carrot, cut into 1/4-inch slices
- 1/2 cup dry white wine
- 3 medium new potatoes, unpeeled and cut into 1-inch pieces
- 1 medium red bell pepper, cut into 1/2-inch dice
- 11/2 cups vegetable broth
- 1 tablespoon minced fresh savory or 1 teaspoon dried

Directions:

1. In a large saucepan, heat the oil over medium heat. Add the onion and carrot, cover, and cook until softened, 7 minutes. Add the wine and cook, uncovered, for 5 minutes. Stir in the potatoes, bell pepper, and broth and bring to a boil. Reduce the heat to medium and simmer for 15 minutes.
2. Add the zucchini, yellow squash, and tomatoes. Season with salt and black pepper to taste, cover, and simmer until the vegetables are tender, 20 to 30 minutes. Stir in the corn, peas, basil, parsley, and savory. Taste, adjusting seasonings if necessary. Simmer to blend flavors, about 10 minutes more. Serve immediately.

Moroccan Vermicelli Vegetable Soup

Preparation Time: 5 minutes

Cooking Time: 35 minutes

Servings: 4 to 6

Ingredients:

- 1 tablespoon olive oil
- 1 small onion, chopped
- 1 large carrot, chopped
- 1 celery rib, chopped
- 3 small zucchini, cut into 1/4-inch dice
- 1 (28-ounce) can diced tomatoes, drained
- 2 tablespoons tomato paste
- 11/2 cups cooked or 1 (15.5-ounce) can chickpeas, drained and rinsed

- 2 teaspoons smoked paprika
- 1 teaspoon ground cumin
- 1 teaspoon za'atar spice (optional)
- 1/4 teaspoon ground cayenne
- 6 cups vegetable broth, homemade (see light vegetable broth) or store-bought, or water
- Salt
- 4 ounces vermicelli
- 2 tablespoons minced fresh cilantro, for garnish

Directions:

1. In a large soup pot, heat the oil over medium heat. Add the onion, carrot, and celery. Cover and cook until softened, about 5 minutes.
2. Stir in the zucchini, tomatoes, tomato paste, chickpeas, paprika, cumin, za'atar, and cayenne.
3. Add the broth and salt to taste. Bring to a boil, then reduce heat to low and simmer, uncovered, until the vegetables are tender, about 30 minutes.
4. Shortly before serving, stir in the vermicelli and cook until the noodles are tender, about 5 minutes. Ladle the soup into bowls, garnish with cilantro, and serve.

Vegetables

Fried Eggs with Kale and Bacon

Preparation Time: 5 minutes
Cooking Time: 15 minutes
Servings: 2
Ingredients:

- 4 slices of turkey bacon, chopped
- 1 bunch of kale, chopped
- 3 oz butter, unsalted
- 2 eggs
- 2 tbsp chopped walnuts
- Seasoning:
- 1/3 tsp salt
- 1/3 tsp ground black pepper

Directions:

1. Take a frying pan, place it over medium heat, add two-third of the butter in it, let it melt, then add kale, switch heat to medium-high level and cook for 4 to 5 minutes until edges have turned golden brown.
2. When done, transfer kale to a plate, set aside until required, add bacon into the pan and cook for 4 minutes until crispy.
3. Return kale into the pan, add nuts, stir until mixed and cook for 2 minutes until thoroughly warmed.
4. Transfer kale into the bowl, add remaining butter into the pan, crack eggs into the pan and fry them for 2 to 3 minutes until cooked to the desired level.
5. Distribute kale between two plates, add fried eggs on the side, sprinkle with salt and black pepper, and then serve.

Eggs with Greens

Preparation Time: 5 minutes
Cooking Time: 10 minutes;
Servings: 2
Ingredients:

- 3 tbsp chopped parsley
- 3 tbsp chopped cilantro
- ¼ tsp cayenne pepper
- 2 eggs
- 1 tbsp butter, unsalted
- Seasoning:
- ¼ tsp salt
- 1/8 tsp ground black pepper

Directions:

1. Take a medium skillet pan, place it over medium-low heat, add butter and wait until it melts.
2. Then add parsley and cilantro, season with salt and black pepper, stir until mixed and cook for 1 minute.
3. Make two space in the pan, crack an egg into each space, and then sprinkle with cayenne pepper, cover the pan with the lid and cook for 2 to 3 minutes until egg yolks have set. Serve.

Spicy Chaffle with Jalapeno

Preparation Time: 5 minutes
Cooking Time: 10 minutes;
Servings: 2
Ingredients:

- 2 tsp coconut flour
- ½ tbsp chopped jalapeno pepper
- 2 tsp cream cheese
- 1 egg
- 2 oz shredded mozzarella cheese
- Seasoning:
- ¼ tsp salt
- 1/8 tsp ground black pepper

Directions:

1. Switch on a mini waffle maker and let it preheat for 5 minutes.
2. Meanwhile, take a medium bowl, place all the ingredients in it and then mix by using an immersion blender until smooth.

3. Ladle the batter evenly into the waffle maker, shut with lid, and let it cook for 3 to 4 minutes until firm and golden brown. Serve.

Pumpkin Smoothie

Preparation Time: 5 minutes
Cooking Time: 0 minutes;
Servings: 2
Ingredients:

- 2 tbsp whipped topping
- 4 tbsp pumpkin puree
- 1 tbsp MCT oil
- ½ cup almond milk, unsweetened
- ½ cup coconut milk, unsweetened
- Seasoning:
- ½ tsp pumpkin pie spice
- 1 ½ cup crushed ice

Directions:

1. Place all the ingredients in the order into a food processor or blender, then pulse for 2 to 3 minutes until smooth.
2. Distribute smoothie between two glasses and then serve.

Bulletproof Tea

Preparation Time: 5 minutes
Cooking Time: 0 minutes
Servings: 2
Ingredients:

- ¼ tsp cinnamon
- 2 cups strong tea
- 2 tbsp coconut oil
- 2 tbsp coconut milk

Directions:

1. Distribute tea between two mugs, add remaining ingredients evenly and then stir until blended.
2. Serve.

Cauliflower and Egg Plate

Preparation Time: 5 minutes
Cooking Time: 12 minutes
Servings: 2
Ingredients:

- 4 oz cauliflower florets, chopped
- 1 jalapeno pepper, sliced
- 2 eggs
- 1 ½ tbsp avocado oil
- Seasoning:
- ¼ tsp salt
- 1/8 tsp ground black pepper

Directions:

1. Take a skillet pan, place it over medium heat, add oil and when hot, add cauliflower florets and jalapeno and then cook for 5 to 7 minutes until tender.
2. Make two spaces in the pan, crack an egg in each space, and then cook for 3 to 4 minutes until eggs have cooked to the desired level. When done, sprinkle salt and black pepper over eggs and then serve.

Butternut Squash and Green Onions with Eggs

Preparation Time: 5 minutes
Cooking Time: 8 minutes;
Servings: 2
Ingredients:

- 4 oz butternut squash pieces
- 1 green onion, sliced
- ½ tbsp butter, unsalted

- 2 tsp grated parmesan cheese
- 2 eggs
- Seasoning:
- ¼ tsp salt
- ¼ tsp ground black pepper
- 1 tsp avocado oil

Directions:
1. Take a skillet pan, place it over medium heat, add butter and oil and when hot, add butternut squash and green onion, season with 1/8 tsp of each salt and black pepper, stir until mixed and cook for 3 to 5 minutes until tender.
2. Make two space in the pan, crack an egg in each space, sprinkle with cheese, season with remaining salt and black pepper, cover with the lid and cook for 2 to 3 minutes until the egg has cooked to the desired level. Serve.

Broccoli, Asparagus and Cheese Frittata

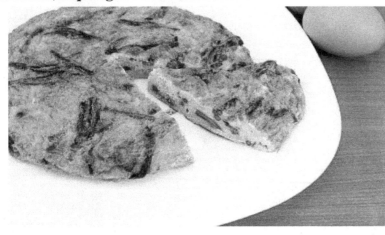

Preparation Time: 5 minutes
Cooking Time: 16 minutes;
Servings: 2
Ingredients:
- ¼ cup chopped broccoli florets
- 1-ounce asparagus spear cuts
- ½ tsp garlic powder
- 2 tbsp whipping cream
- 2 eggs
- 2 tsp tbsp avocado oil
- 1/8 tsp salt
- 1/8 tsp ground black pepper

Directions:
1. Turn on the oven, then set it to 350 degrees F and let it preheat.
2. Take a medium bowl, crack eggs in it, add salt, black pepper and cream, whisk until combined and then stir in cheese, set aside until required.
3. Take a medium skillet pan, place it over medium heat, add oil and when hot, add broccoli florets and asparagus, sprinkle with garlic powder, stir until mixed and cook for 3 to 4 minutes until tender.
4. Spread the vegetables evenly in the pan, pour egg mixture over them and cook for 1 to 2 minutes until the mixture begins.
5. Transfer the pan into the oven and then cook for 10 to 12 minutes until frittata has cooked and the top has turned golden brown. When done, cut the frittata into slices and then serve.

Broccoli and Egg Plate

Preparation Time: 5 minutes
Cooking Time: 5 minutes;
Servings: 2
Ingredients:
- 3 oz broccoli florets, chopped
- 2 eggs
- 1 tbsp avocado oil
- ¼ tsp salt
- 1/8 tsp ground black pepper

Directions:
1. Take a bowl, place broccoli florets in it, cover with a plastic wrap, microwave for 2 minutes, and then drain well.
2. Take a medium skillet pan, place it over medium heat, add oil and when hot, add broccoli florets and cook for 2 minutes until golden brown.

3. Spread broccoli florets evenly in the pan crack eggs in the pan, sprinkle with salt and black pepper, cover with the lid and cook for 2 to 3 minutes until eggs have cooked to the desired level.
4. Serve.

Radish with Fried Eggs

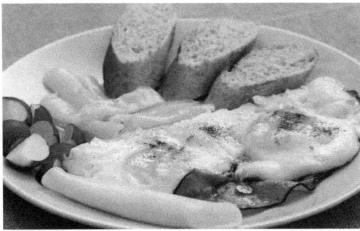

Preparation Time: 5 minutes
Cooking Time: 10 minutes;
Servings: 2
Ingredients:
- ½ bunch of radish, diced
- ½ tsp garlic powder
- 1 tbsp butter
- 1 tbsp avocado oil
- 2 eggs
- Seasoning:
- 1/3 tsp salt
- ¼ tsp ground black pepper

Directions:
1. Take a medium skillet pan, place it over medium heat, add butter. When it melts, add radish, sprinkle with garlic powder and ¼ tsp salt and cook for 5 minutes until tender.
2. Distribute radish between two plates, then return pan over medium heat, add oil and hot, crack eggs in it and fry for 2 to 3 minutes until cooked to the desired level.
3. Add eggs to the radish and then serve.

Sunny Side Up Eggs on Creamed Spinach

Preparation Time: 5 minutes
Cooking Time: 10 minutes;
Servings: 2
Ingredients:
- 4 oz of spinach leaves
- 1 tbsp mustard paste
- 4 tbsp whipping cream
- 2 eggs
- Seasoning:
- ¼ tsp salt
- ¼ tsp ground black pepper
- ½ tsp dried thyme
- 1 tbsp avocado oil

Directions:
1. Take a medium skillet pan, place it over high heat, pour in water to cover its bottom, then add spinach, toss until mixed and cook for 2 minutes until spinach wilts.
2. Then drain the spinach by passing it through a sieve placed on a bowl and set it aside.
3. Take a medium saucepan, place it over medium heat, add spinach, mustard, thyme, and cream, stir until mixed and cook for 2 minutes.
4. Then sprinkle black pepper over spinach, stir until mixed and remove the pan from heat.
5. Take a medium skillet pan, place it over medium-high heat, add oil and when hot, crack eggs in it and fry for 3 to 4 minutes until eggs have cooked to the desired level.
6. Divide spinach mixture evenly between two plates, top with a fried egg and then serve.

Creamy Kale Baked Eggs

Preparation Time: 10 minutes
Cooking Time: 20 minutes
Servings: 2
Ingredients:

- 1 bunch of kale, chopped
- 1-ounce grape tomatoes, halved
- 3 tbsp whipping cream
- 2 tbsp sour cream
- 2 eggs
- Seasoning:
- ½ tsp salt
- ½ tsp ground black pepper
- ½ tsp Italian seasoning
- 1 ½ tbsp butter, unsalted

Directions:

1. Turn on the oven, then set it to 400 degrees F and let it preheat.
2. Meanwhile, take a medium skillet pan, place butter in it, add butter and when it melts, add kale and cook for 2 minutes until wilted
3. Add Italian seasoning, 1/3 tsp each of salt and black pepper, cream and sour cream, then stir until mixed and cook for2 minutes until cheese has melted and the kale has thickened slightly.
4. Take two ramekins, divide creamed kale evenly between them, then top with cherry tomatoes and carefully crack an egg into each ramekin.
5. Sprinkle remaining salt and black pepper on eggs and then bake for 15 minutes until eggs have cooked completely. Serve.

Veggie Fritters

Preparation Time: 10 minutes
Cooking Time: 10 minutes
Servings: 4
Ingredients:

- 2 garlic cloves, minced
- 2 yellow onions, chopped
- 4 scallions, chopped
- 2 carrots, grated
- 2 teaspoons cumin, ground
- ½ teaspoon turmeric powder
- Salt and black pepper to the taste
- ¼ teaspoon coriander, ground
- 2 tablespoons parsley, chopped
- ¼ teaspoon lemon juice
- ½ cup almond flour
- 2 beets, peeled and grated
- 2 eggs, whisked
- ¼ cup tapioca flour
- 3 tablespoons olive oil

Directions:

1. In a bowl, combine the garlic with the onions, scallions and the rest of the ingredients except the oil, stir well and shape medium fritters out of this mix.
2. Heat oil in a pan over medium-high heat, add the fritters, cook for 5 minutes on each side, arrange on a platter and serve.

Salad Recipes

Southwest Style Salad

Preparation Time: 25 minutes

Cooking Time: 15 minutes

Servings: 3

Ingredients:

- ½ cup dry black beans
- ½ cup dry chickpeas
- 1/3 cup purple onion, diced
- 1 red bell pepper, pitted, sliced

- 4 cups mixed greens, fresh or frozen, chopped
- 1 cup cherry tomatoes, halved or quartered
- 1 medium avocado, peeled, pitted, and cubed
- 1 cup sweet kernel corn, canned, drained
- ½ tsp. chili powder
- ¼ tsp. cumin
- ¼ tsp Salt
- ¼ tsp pepper
- 2 tsp. olive oil
- 1 tbsp. vinegar

Directions:

1. Take a pot and bring the water to a boil. Season with salt and add beans and chickpeas. Cook them on medium for 15 minutes.
2. Put all of the ingredients into a large bowl.
3. Toss the mix of veggies and spices until combined thoroughly.
4. Store, or serve chilled with some olive oil and vinegar on top!

Shaved Brussel Sprout Salad

Preparation Time: 40 minutes

Cooking Time: 15 minutes

Servings: 4

Ingredients:

DRESSING:

- 1 tbsp. brown mustard
- 1 tbsp. maple syrup
- 2 tbsp. apple cider vinegar
- 2 tbsp. extra virgin olive oil
- ½ tbsp. garlic minced

SALAD:

- ½ cup dry red kidney beans
- ¼ cup dry chickpeas
- 2 cups Brussel sprouts
- 1 cup purple onion
- 1 small sour apple
- ½ cup slivered almonds, crushed
- ½ cup walnuts, crushed
- ½ cup cranberries, dried
- ¼ tsp Salt
- ¼ tsp pepper

Directions:

1. Take a pot and bring the water to a boil. Season with salt and add beans. Cook them on medium for 15 minutes.
2. Combine all dressing ingredients in a bowl and stir well until combined.
3. Refrigerate the dressing for up to one hour before serving.
4. Using a grater, mandolin, or knife to slice each Brussel sprout thinly. Repeat this with the apple and onion.
5. Take a large bowl to mix the chickpeas, beans, sprouts, apples, onions, cranberries, and nuts.
6. Drizzle the cold dressing over the salad to coat. Serve with salt and pepper to taste!

Colorful Protein Power Salad

Preparation Time: 30 minutes

Cooking Time: 20 minutes

Servings: 2

Ingredients:

- ½ cup dry quinoa
- 2 cups dry navy beans
- 1 green onion, chopped

- 2 tsp. garlic, minced
- 3 cups green or purple cabbage, chopped
- 4 cups kale, fresh or frozen, chopped
- 1 cup shredded carrot, chopped
- 2 tbsp. extra virgin olive oil
- 1 tsp. lemon juice
- ¼ tsp Salt
- ¼ tsp pepper

Directions:
1. Take a pot and bring the water to a boil. Season with salt and add quinoa. Cook them on medium for 5 minutes
2. Take a pot and bring the water to a boil. Season with salt and add beans. Cook them on medium for 15 minutes
3. Heat 1 tablespoon of the olive oil in a frying pan over medium heat.
4. Add the chopped green onion, garlic, and cabbage, and sauté for 2-3 minutes.
5. Add the kale, the remaining 1 tablespoon of olive oil, and salt. Lower the heat and cover until the greens have wilted, around 5 minutes. Remove the pan from the stove and set aside.
6. Take a large bowl and mix the remaining ingredients with the kale and cabbage mixture once it has cooled down. Add more salt and pepper to taste. Mix until everything is distributed evenly. Serve topped with a dressing.

Edamame and Ginger Citrus Salad

Preparation Time: 25 minutes
Cooking Time: 15 minutes
 Servings: 3
Ingredients:
DRESSING:

- ¼ cup orange juice
- 1 tsp. lime juice
- ½ tbsp. maple syrup
- ½ tsp. ginger, finely minced
- ½ tbsp. sesame oil

SALAD:
- ½ cup dry green lentils
- 2 cups carrots, shredded
- 4 cups kale, fresh or frozen, chopped
- 1 cup edamame, shelled
- 1 tablespoon roasted sesame seeds
- 2 tsp. mint, chopped
- Salt and pepper to taste
- 1 small avocado, peeled, pitted, diced

Directions:
1. Take a pot and bring the water to a boil. Season with salt and add lentils. Cook them on medium for 15 minutes.
2. Combine the orange and lime juices, maple syrup, and ginger in a small bowl. Mix with a whisk while slowly adding the sesame oil. Add the cooked lentils, carrots, kale, edamame, sesame seeds, and mint to a large bowl.
3. Add the dressing and stir well until all the ingredients are coated evenly.
4. Serve topped with avocado and an additional sprinkle of mint.

Taco Tempeh Salad

Preparation Time: 25 minutes
Cooking Time: 0 minutes
Servings: 3
Ingredients:
- 1 cup dry black beans
- 1 8-oz. package tempeh
- 1 tbsp. lime or lemon juice
- 2 tbsp. extra virgin olive oil
- 1 tsp. maple syrup
- ½ tsp. chili powder
- ¼ tsp. cumin
- ¼ tsp. paprika
- 1 large bunch of kale, fresh or frozen, chopped
- 1 large avocado, peeled, pitted, diced
- ½ cup salsa
- ¼ tsp Salt
- ¼ tsp pepper

Directions:
1. Take a pot and bring the water to a boil. Season with salt and add beans. Cook them on medium for 15 minutes

2. Cut the tempeh into ¼-inch cubes, place in a bowl, and then add the lime or lemon juice, 1 tablespoon of olive oil, maple syrup, chili powder, cumin, and paprika.
3. Stir well and let the tempeh marinate in the fridge for at least 1 hour, up to 12 hours.
4. Heat the remaining 1 tablespoon of olive oil in a frying pan over medium heat.
5. Add the marinated tempeh mixture and cook until brown and crispy on both sides, around 10 minutes.
6. Put the chopped kale in a bowl with the cooked beans and prepared tempeh.
7. Store, or serve the salad immediately, topped with salsa, avocado, and salt and pepper to taste.

Lebanese Potato Salad
Preparation Time: 5 minutes
Cooking Time: 10 minutes
Servings: 4
Ingredients:
- 1-pound Russet potatoes
- 1 ½ tablespoons extra virgin olive oil
- 2 scallions, thinly sliced
- Freshly ground pepper to taste
- 2 tablespoons lemon juice
- ¼ teaspoon salt or to taste
- 2 tablespoons fresh mint leaves, chopped

Directions:
1. Place a saucepan half filled with water over medium heat. Add salt and potatoes and cook for 10 minutes until tender. Drain the potatoes and place in a bowl of cold water. When cool enough to handle, peel and cube the potatoes. Place in a bowl.

To make dressing:
2. Add oil, lemon juice, salt and pepper in a bowl and whisk well. Drizzle dressing over the potatoes. Toss well.
3. Add scallions and mint and toss well.
4. Divide into 4 plates and serve.

Chickpea and Spinach Salad
Preparation Time: 5 minutes
Cooking Time: 0 minutes
Servings: 4
Ingredients:
- 2 cans (14.5 ounces each) chickpeas, drained, rinsed
- 7 ounces vegan feta cheese, crumbled or chopped
- 1 tablespoon lemon juice
- 1/3 -½ cup olive oil
- ½ teaspoon salt or to taste
- 4-6 cups spinach, torn
- ½ cup raisins
- 2 tablespoons honey
- 1-2 teaspoons ground cumin
- 1 teaspoon chili flakes

Directions:
1. Add cheese, chickpeas and spinach into a large bowl.
2. To make dressing: Add rest of the ingredients into another bowl and mix well.
3. Pour dressing over the salad. Toss well and serve.

Tempeh "Chicken" Salad
Preparation Time: 10 minutes
Cooking Time: 0 minutes
Servings: 2
Ingredients:
- 4 tablespoons light mayonnaise
- 2 scallions, sliced
- Pepper to taste

- 4 cups mixed salad greens
- 4 teaspoons white miso
- 2 tablespoons chopped fresh dill
- 1 ½ cups crumbled tempeh
- 1 cup sliced grape tomatoes

Directions:

To make dressing:
1. Add mayonnaise, scallions, miso, dill and pepper into a bowl and whisk well.
2. Add tempeh and fold gently.

To serve:
3. Divide the greens into 4 plates. Divide the tempeh among the plates. Top with tomatoes and serve.

Spinach and Dill Pasta Salad

Preparation Time: 5 minutes
Cooking Time: 0 minutes
Servings: 4
Ingredients:
FOR SALAD:

- 3 cups cooked whole-wheat fusilli
- 2 cups cherry tomatoes, halved
- ½ cup vegan cheese, shredded
- 4 cups spinach, chopped
- 2 cups edamame, thawed
- 1 large red onion, finely chopped

FOR DRESSING:
- 2 tablespoons white wine vinegar
- ½ teaspoon dried dill
- 2 tablespoons extra-virgin olive oil
- Salt to taste
- Pepper to taste

Directions:

To make dressing:
1. Add all the ingredients for dressing into a bowl and whisk well. Set aside for a while for the flavors to set in.

To make salad:
2. Add all the ingredients of the salad in a bowl. Toss well.
3. Drizzle dressing on top. Toss well.
4. Divide into 4 plates and serve.

Italian Veggie Salad

Preparation Time: 10 minutes
Cooking Time: 0 minutes
Servings: 8
Ingredients:
FOR SALAD:

- 1 cup fresh baby carrots, quartered lengthwise
- 1 celery rib, sliced
- 3 large mushrooms, thinly sliced
- 1 cup cauliflower florets, bite sized, blanched
- 1 cup broccoli florets, blanched
- 1 cup thinly sliced radish
- 4-5 ounces hearts of romaine salad mix to serve

FOR DRESSING:
- ½ package Italian salad dressing mix
- 3 tablespoons white vinegar
- 3 tablespoons water
- 3 tablespoons olive oil
- 3-4 pepperoncino, chopped

Directions:

To make salad:
1. Add all the ingredients of the salad except hearts of romaine to a bowl and toss.

To make dressing:
2. Add all the ingredients of the dressing in a small bowl. Whisk well.
3. Pour dressing over salad and toss well. Refrigerate for a couple of hours.

4. Place romaine in a large bowl. Place the chilled salad over it and serve.

Wasabi Tuna Asian Salad

Preparation Time: 30 minutes
Cooking Time: 10 minutes
Servings: 1
Ingredients:

- Lime juice (1 teaspoon)
- Non-stick cooking spray
- Pepper/dash of salt
- Wasabi paste (1 teaspoon)
- Olive oil (2 teaspoons)
- Chopped or shredded cucumbers (1/2 cup)
- Bok Choy stalks (1 cup)
- Raw tuna steak (8 oz.)

Directions:

1. Fish: preheat your skillet to medium heat. Mix your wasabi and lime juice; coat the tuna steaks.
2. Use a non-stick cooking spray on your skillet for 10 seconds.
3. Put your tuna steaks on the skillet and cook over medium heat until you get the desired doneness.
4. Salad: Slice the cucumber into match-stick tiny sizes. Cut the bok Choy into minute pieces. Toss gently with pepper, salt, and olive oil if you want. Enjoy!

Lemon Greek Salad

Preparation Time: 25 minutes
Cooking Time: 25 minutes
Servings: 1
Ingredients:

- Chicken breast (140 oz)
- Chopped cucumber (1 cup)
- Chopped orange/red bell pepper (1 cup)
- Wedged/sliced/chopped tomatoes (1 cup)
- Chopped olives (1/4 cup)
- Fresh parsley (2 tablespoons), finely chopped.
- Finely chopped red onion (2 tablespoons)
- Lemon juice (5 teaspoons)
- Olive oil (1 teaspoon)
- Minced garlic (1 clove)

Directions:

1. Preheat your grill to medium heat.
2. Grill the chicken and cook on each side until the chicken is no longer pink or for 5 minutes.
3. Cut the chicken into tiny pieces. In your serving bowl, mix garlic, olives, and parsley. Whisk in olive oil (1 teaspoon) and lemon juice (4 teaspoons). Add onion, tomatoes, bell pepper, and cucumber.
4. Toss gently. Coat the ingredients with dressing. Add another teaspoon of lemon juice to taste. Divide the salad into two servings and put 6oz chicken on top of each salad. Enjoy!

Broccoli Salad

Preparation Time: 5 minutes
Cooking Time: 25 minutes
Servings: 1
Ingredients:

- 1/3 tablespoons sherry vinegar
- 1/24 cup olive oil
- 1/3 teaspoons fresh thyme, chopped
- 1/6 teaspoon Dijon mustard
- 1/6 teaspoon honey
- Salt to taste
- 1 1/3 cups broccoli florets
- 1/3 red onions
- 1/12 cup parmesan cheese shaved
- 1/24 cup pecans

Directions:

1. Mix the sherry vinegar, olive oil, thyme, mustard, honey, and salt in a bowl.
2. In a serving bowl, blend the broccoli florets and onions.

3. Drizzle the dressing on top.
4. Sprinkle with the pecans and parmesan cheese before serving.

Potato Carrot Salad

Preparation Time: 4 hours 15 minutes

Cooking Time: 10 minutes

Servings: 1

Ingredients:

- Water
- 1 potato, sliced into cubes
- 1/2 carrots, cut into cubes
- 1/6 tablespoon milk
- 1/6 tablespoon Dijon mustard
- 1/24 cup mayonnaise
- Pepper to taste
- 1/3 teaspoons fresh thyme, chopped
- 1/6 stalk celery, chopped
- 1/6 scallions, chopped
- 1/6 slice turkey bacon, cooked crispy and crumbled

Directions:

1. Fill your pot with water and place it over medium-high heat.
2. Boil the potatoes and carrots for 10 to 12 minutes or until tender. Drain and let cool.
3. In a bowl, mix the milk, mustard, mayonnaise, pepper, and thyme.
4. Stir in the potatoes, carrots, and celery.
5. Coat evenly with the sauce.
6. Cover and refrigerate for 4 hours.
7. Top with the scallions and turkey bacon bits before serving.

Marinated Veggie Salad

Preparation Time: 4 hours and 30 minutes

Cooking Time: 3 minutes

Servings: 1

Ingredients:

- 1 zucchini, sliced
- 4 tomatoes, sliced into wedges
- ¼ cup red onion, sliced thinly
- 1 green bell pepper, sliced
- 2 tablespoons fresh parsley, chopped
- 2 tablespoons red-wine vinegar
- 2 tablespoons olive oil
- 1 clove garlic, minced
- 1 teaspoon dried basil
- 2 tablespoons water
- Pine nuts, toasted and chopped

Directions:

1. In a bowl, combine the zucchini, tomatoes, red onion, green bell pepper, and parsley.
2. Pour the vinegar and oil into a glass jar with a lid. Add the garlic, basil, and water. Seal the jar and stir well to combine. Pour the dressing into the vegetable mixture. Cover the bowl.
3. Marinate in the refrigerator for 4 hours.
4. Garnish with the pine nuts before serving.

Mediterranean Salad

Preparation Time: 20 minutes

Cooking Time: 5 minutes

Servings: 1

Ingredients:

- 1 teaspoon balsamic vinegar
- 1/2 tablespoon basil pesto
- 1/2 cup lettuce
- 1/8 cup broccoli florets, chopped
- 1/8 cup zucchini, chopped

- 1/8 cup tomato, chopped
- 1/8 cup yellow bell pepper, chopped
- 1/2 tablespoons feta cheese, crumbled

Directions:
1. Arrange the lettuce on a serving platter. Top with the broccoli, zucchini, tomato, and bell pepper.
2. In a bowl, mix the vinegar and pesto.
3. Drizzle the dressing on top. Sprinkle the feta cheese and serve.

Potato Tuna Salad
Preparation Time: 4 hours and 20 minutes
Cooking Time: 10 minutes
Servings: 1
Ingredients:
- 1 potato, peeled and sliced into cubes
- 1/12 cup plain yogurt
- 1/12 cup mayonnaise
- 1/6 clove garlic, crushed and minced
- 1/6 tablespoon almond milk
- 1/6 tablespoon fresh dill, chopped
- ½ teaspoon lemon zest
- Salt to taste
- 1 cup cucumber, chopped
- ¼ cup scallions, chopped
- ¼ cup radishes, chopped
- (9 oz) canned tuna flakes
- 1/2 hard-boiled eggs, chopped
- 1 cups lettuce, chopped

Directions:
1. Fill your pot with water, add the potatoes and boil for 15 minutes. Drain and let cool.
2. In a bowl, mix the yogurt, mayo, garlic, almond milk, fresh dill, lemon zest, and salt.
3. Stir in the potatoes, tuna flakes, and eggs. Mix well.
4. Chill in the refrigerator for 4 hours. Stir in the shredded lettuce before serving.

High Protein Salad
Preparation Time: 5 minutes
Cooking Time: 5 minutes
Servings: 1
Ingredients:
SALAD:
- 1(15 oz) can green kidney beans
- 1/4 tablespoon capers
- 1/4 handfuls arugula
- 1(15 oz) can lentils

DRESSING:
- 1/1 tablespoon caper brine
- 1/1 tablespoon tamari
- 1/1 tablespoon balsamic vinegar
- 2/2 tablespoon peanut butter
- 2/2 tablespoon hot sauce
- 2/1 tablespoon tahini

Directions:
For the dressing:
1. In a bowl, stir all the ingredients until they come together to form a smooth dressing.
For the salad:
2. Mix the beans, arugula, capers, and lentils. Top with the dressing and serve.

Rice and Veggie Bowl
Preparation Time: 5 minutes
Cooking Time: 15 minutes
Servings: 1
Ingredients:
- 1/3 tablespoon coconut oil
- 1/2 teaspoon ground cumin
- 1/2 teaspoon ground turmeric
- 1/3 teaspoon chili powder

- 1 red bell pepper, chopped
- 1/2 tablespoon tomato paste
- 1 bunch of broccoli, cut into bite-sized florets with short stems
- 1/2 teaspoon salt, to taste
- 1 large red onion, sliced
- 1/2 garlic cloves, minced
- 1/2 head of cauliflower, sliced into bite-sized florets
- 1/2 cups cooked rice
- Newly ground black pepper to taste

Directions:

1. Start with warming up the coconut oil over medium-high heat.
2. Stir in the turmeric, cumin, chili powder, salt, and tomato paste.
3. Cook the content for 1 minute. Stir repeatedly until the spices are fragrant.
4. Add the garlic and onion. Fry for 2 to 3 minutes until the onions are softened.
5. Add the broccoli, cauliflower, and bell pepper. Cover then cook for 3 to 4 minutes and stir occasionally.
6. Add the cooked rice. Stir so it will combine well with the vegetables. Cook for 2 to 3 minutes. Stir until the rice is warm. Check the seasoning and change to taste if desired.
7. Lessen the heat and cook on low for 2 to 3 more minutes so the flavors will meld.
8. Serve with freshly ground black pepper.

Squash Black Bean Bowl

Preparation Time: 5 minutes
Cooking Time: 30 minutes
Servings: 1
Ingredients:

- 1 large spaghetti squash, halved,
- 1/3 cup water (or 2 tablespoon olive oil, rubbed on the inside of squash)

BLACK BEAN FILLING:

- 1/2 (15 oz) can of black beans, emptied and rinsed
- 1/2 cup fire-roasted corn (or frozen sweet corn)
- 1/2 cup thinly sliced red cabbage
- 1/2 tablespoon chopped green onion, green and white parts
- ¼ cup chopped fresh coriander
- ½ lime, juiced or to taste
- Pepper and salt, to taste

AVOCADO MASH:

- One ripe avocado, mashed
- ½ lime, juiced or to taste
- ¼ teaspoon cumin
- Pepper and pinch of sea salt

Directions:

1. Preheat the oven to 400°F.
2. Chop the squash in part and scoop out the seeds with a spoon, like a pumpkin.
3. Fill the roasting pan with 1/3 cup of water. Lay the squash, cut side down, in the pan. Bake for 30 minutes until soft and tender.
4. While this is baking, mix all the ingredients for the black bean filling in a medium-sized bowl.
5. In a small dish, crush the avocado and blend in the ingredients for the avocado mash.
6. Eliminate the squash from the oven and let it cool for 5 minutes. Scrape the squash with a fork so that it looks like spaghetti noodles. Then, fill it with black bean filling and top with avocado mash.
7. Serve and enjoy.

Pea Salad

Preparation Time: 40 minutes
Cooking Time: 0 minutes
Servings: 1

Ingredients:

- 1/2 cup chickpeas, rinsed and drained
- 1/2 cups peas, divided

- Salt to taste
- 1 tablespoon olive oil
- ½ cup buttermilk
- Pepper to taste

- 2 cups pea greens
- 1/2 carrots shaved
- 1/4 cup snow peas, trimmed

Directions:

1. Add the chickpeas, salt and half of the peas in your food processor. Pulse until smooth. Set aside.
2. In a bowl, toss the remaining peas in oil, milk, salt, and pepper.
3. Transfer the mixture to your food processor. Process until pureed. Transfer this mixture to a bowl.
4. Arrange the pea greens on a serving plate. Top with the shaved carrots and snow peas.
5. Stir in the pea and milk dressing. Serve with the reserved chickpea hummus.

Snap Pea Salad

Preparation Time: 1 hour
Cooking Time: 0 minutes
Servings: 1
Ingredients:

- 1/2 tablespoons mayonnaise
- ¾ teaspoon celery seed

- ¼ cup cider vinegar
- 1/2 teaspoon yellow mustard
- 1/2 tablespoon sugar
- Salt and pepper to taste
- 1 oz. radishes, sliced thinly
- 2 oz. sugar snap peas, sliced thinly

Directions:

1. In a bowl, combine the mayonnaise, celery seeds, vinegar, mustard, sugar, salt, and pepper.
2. Stir in the radishes and snap peas. Refrigerate for 30 minutes. Serve.

Cucumber Tomato Chopped Salad

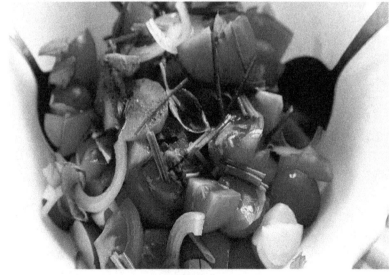

Preparation Time: 15 minutes
Cooking Time: 0 minutes
Servings: 1
Ingredients:

- 1/4 cup light mayonnaise
- 1/2 tablespoon lemon juice
- 1/2 tablespoon fresh dill, chopped
- 1/2 tablespoon chive, chopped
- 1/4 cup feta cheese, crumbled
- Salt and pepper to taste
- 1/2 red onion, chopped
- 1/2 cucumber, diced
- 1/2 radish, diced
- 1 tomato, diced
- Chives, chopped

Directions:

1. Combine the mayonnaise, lemon juice, fresh dill, chives, feta cheese, salt, and pepper in a bowl. Mix well.
2. Stir in the onion, cucumber, radish, and tomatoes.
3. Coat evenly. Garnish with the chopped chives and serve!

Zucchini Pasta Salad

Preparation Time: 4 minutes

Cooking Time: 0 minutes

Servings: 1

Ingredients:

- 1 tablespoon olive oil
- 1/2 teaspoons dijon mustard
- 1/3 tablespoons red-wine vinegar
- 1/2 clove garlic, grated
- 2 tablespoons fresh oregano, chopped
- 1/2 shallot, chopped
- ¼ teaspoon red pepper flakes
- 4 oz. zucchini noodles
- ¼ cup Kalamata olives pitted
- 1 cups cherry tomato, sliced in half
- ¾ cup parmesan cheese shaved

Directions:

1. Mix the olive oil, Dijon mustard, red wine vinegar, garlic, oregano, shallot, and red pepper flakes in a bowl.
2. Stir in the zucchini noodles.
3. Sprinkle on top the olives, tomatoes, and parmesan cheese.

Egg Avocado Salad

Preparation Time: 10 minutes

Cooking Time: 0 minutes

Servings: 1

Ingredients:

- 1/2 avocado
- 1 hard-boiled egg, peeled and chopped
- 1/4 tablespoon mayonnaise
- 1/4 tablespoons freshly squeezed lemon juice
- ¼ cup celery, chopped
- 1/2 tablespoons chives, chopped
- Salt and pepper to taste

Directions:

1. Add the avocado to a large bowl. Mash the avocado using a fork.
2. Stir in the egg and mash the eggs.
3. Add the mayonnaise, lemon juice, celery, chives, salt, and pepper.
4. Chill in the refrigerator for at least 2o to 30 minutes before serving.

Olives and Cheese Stuffed Tomatoes

Preparation Time: 10 minutes

Cooking Time: 0 minutes

Servings: 24

Ingredients:

- 24 cherry tomatoes, top cut off and insides scooped out
- 2 tablespoons olive oil
- ¼ teaspoon red pepper flakes
- ½ cup feta cheese, crumbled
- 2 tablespoons black olive paste
- ¼ cup mint, torn

Directions:

1. In a bowl, mix the olives paste with the rest of the ingredients except the cherry tomatoes and whisk well.
2. Stuff the cherry tomatoes with this mix, arrange them all on a platter and serve as an appetizer.

Seafood

Baked Cod Crusted with Herbs

Preparation Time: 5 minutes

Cooking Time: 10 minutes

Servings: 4

Ingredients:

- ¼ cup honey
- ¼ teaspoon salt
- ½ cup panko
- ½ teaspoon pepper
- 1 tablespoon extra-virgin olive oil
- 1 tablespoon lemon juice
- 1 teaspoon dried basil
- 1 teaspoon dried parsley
- 1 teaspoon rosemary
- 4 pieces of 4-oz cod fillets

Directions:

1. With olive oil, grease a 9 x 13-inch baking pan and preheat oven to 375°F.
2. In a zip top bag mix panko, rosemary, salt, pepper, parsley and basil.
3. Evenly spread cod fillets in prepped dish and drizzle with lemon juice. Then brush the fillets with honey on all sides. Discard remaining honey if any. Then evenly divide the panko mixture on top of cod fillets.
4. Pop in the oven and bake for ten minutes or until fish is cooked. Serve and enjoy.

Coconut Salsa on Chipotle Fish Tacos

Preparation Time: 10 minutes

Cooking Time: 10 minutes

Servings: 4

Ingredients:

- ¼ cup chopped fresh cilantro
- ½ cup seeded and finely chopped plum tomato
- 1 cup peeled and finely chopped mango
- 1 lime cut into wedges
- 1 tablespoon chipotle Chile powder
- 1 tablespoon safflower oil
- 1/3 cup finely chopped red onion
- 10 tablespoon fresh lime juice, divided
- 4 6-oz boneless, skinless cod fillets
- 5 tablespoon dried unsweetened shredded coconut
- 8 pcs of 6-inch tortillas, heated

Directions:

1. Whisk well Chile powder, oil, and 4 tablespoon lime juice in a glass baking dish. Add cod and marinate for 12 – 15 minutes. Turning once halfway through the marinating time.
2. Make the salsa by mixing coconut, 6 tablespoon lime juice, cilantro, onions, tomatoes and mangoes in a medium bowl. Set aside.
3. On high, heat a grill pan. Place cod and grill for four minutes per side turning only once. Once cooked, slice cod into large flakes and evenly divide onto tortilla. Divide salsa on top of cod and serve with a side of lime wedges.

Creamy Bacon-Fish Chowder

Preparation Time: 10 minutes

Cooking Time: 30 minutes

Servings: 8

Ingredients:

- 1 1/2 lbs. cod
- 1 1/2 teaspoon dried thyme
- 1 large onion, chopped
- 1 medium carrot, coarsely chopped
- 1 tablespoon butter, cut into small pieces
- 1 teaspoon salt, divided
- 3 1/2 cups baking potato, peeled and cubed
- 3 slices uncooked bacon
- 3/4 teaspoon ground black pepper, divided
- 4 1/2 cups water
- 4 bay leaves
- 4 cups 2% reduced-fat milk

Directions:

1. In a large skillet, add the water and bay leaves and let it simmer. Add the fish. Cover and let it simmer some more until the flesh flakes easily with fork. Remove the fish from the skillet and cut into large pieces. Set aside the cooking liquid.
2. Place Dutch oven in medium heat and cook the bacon until crisp. Remove the bacon and reserve the bacon drippings. Crush the bacon and set aside.
3. Stir potato, onion and carrot in the pan with the bacon drippings, cook over medium heat for 10 minutes. Add the cooking liquid, bay leaves, 1/2 teaspoon salt, 1/4 teaspoon pepper and thyme, let it boil. Lower the heat and let simmer for 11 minutes. Add the milk and butter, simmer until the potatoes becomes tender, but do not boil. Add the fish, 1/2 teaspoon salt, 1/2 teaspoon pepper. Remove the bay leaves.
4. Serve sprinkled with the crushed bacon.

Crazy Saganaki Shrimp

Preparation Time: 10 minutes
Cooking Time: 10 minutes
Servings: 4
Ingredients:

- ¼ teaspoon salt
- ½ cup Chardonnay
- ½ cup crumbled Greek feta cheese
- 1 medium bulb. fennel, cored and finely chopped
- 1 small Chile pepper, seeded and minced
- 1 tablespoon extra-virgin olive oil
- 12 jumbo shrimps, deveined with tails left on
- 2 tablespoon lemon juice, divided
- 5 scallions sliced thinly
- Pepper to taste

Directions:

1. In medium bowl, mix salt, lemon juice and shrimp.
2. On medium fire, place a saganaki pan (or large nonstick saucepan) and heat oil.
3. Sauté Chile pepper, scallions, and fennel for 4 minutes or until starting to brown and is already soft. Add wine and sauté for another minute. Place shrimps on top of fennel, cover and cook for 4 minutes or until shrimps are pink.
4. Remove just the shrimp and transfer to a plate.
5. Add pepper, feta and 1 tablespoon lemon juice to pan and cook for a minute or until cheese begins to melt.
6. To serve, place cheese and fennel mixture on a serving plate and top with shrimps.

Cajun Garlic Shrimp Noodle Bowl

Preparation Time: 10 minutes
Cooking Time: 15 minutes
Servings: 2
Ingredients:

- ½ teaspoon salt
- 1 onion, sliced
- 1 red pepper, sliced
- 1 tablespoon butter
- 1 teaspoon garlic granules
- 1 teaspoon onion powder
- 1 teaspoon paprika
- 2 large zucchinis, cut into noodle strips
- 20 jumbo shrimps, shells removed and deveined
- 3 cloves garlic, minced
- 3 tablespoon ghee
- A dash of cayenne pepper
- A dash of red pepper flakes

Directions:

1. Prepare the Cajun seasoning by mixing the onion powder, garlic granules, pepper flakes, cayenne pepper, paprika and salt. Toss in the shrimp to coat in the seasoning.
2. In a skillet, heat the ghee and sauté the garlic, then add red pepper and onions and sauté for 4 minutes.

3. Add the Cajun shrimp and cook until opaque. Set aside.
4. In another pan, heat the butter and sauté the zucchini noodles for three minutes.
5. Assemble by the placing the Cajun shrimps on top of the zucchini noodles.

Cucumber-Basil Salsa on Halibut Pouches

Preparation Time: 10 minutes
Cooking Time: 17 minutes
Servings: 4
Ingredients:

- 1 lime, thinly sliced into 8 pieces
- 2 cups mustard greens, stems removed
- 2 teaspoon olive oil
- 4 – 5 radishes trimmed and quartered
- 4 4-oz skinless halibut filets
- 4 large fresh basil leaves
- Cayenne pepper to taste – optional
- Pepper and salt to taste

SALSA:

- 1 ½ cups diced cucumber
- 1 ½ finely chopped fresh basil leaves
- 2 teaspoon fresh lime juice
- Pepper and salt to taste

Directions:

1. Preheat oven to 400°F. Prepare parchment papers by making 4 pieces of 15 x 12-inch rectangles. Lengthwise, fold in half and unfold pieces on the table.
2. Season halibut fillets with pepper, salt and pepper. Just to the right of the fold, place ½ cup of mustard greens. Add a basil leaf on center of mustard greens and topped with 1 lime slice. Around the greens, layer ¼ of the radishes. Drizzle with ½ teaspoon of oil, season with pepper and salt. Top it with a slice of halibut fillet.
3. Just as you would make a calzone, fold parchment paper over your filling and crimp the edges of the parchment paper beginning from one end to the other end. To seal the end of the crimped parchment paper, pinch it.
4. Repeat process to remaining ingredients until you have 4 pieces of parchment papers filled with halibut and greens. Place pouches in a pan and bake in the oven until halibut is flaky, around 15 to 17 minutes.
5. While waiting for halibut pouches to cook, make your salsa by mixing all salsa ingredients in a medium bowl.
6. Once halibut is cooked, remove from oven and make a tear on top. Be careful of the steam as it is very hot. Equally divide salsa and spoon ¼ of salsa on top of halibut through the slit you have created.

Curry Salmon with Mustard

Preparation Time: 10 minutes
Cooking Time: 8 minutes
Servings: 4
Ingredients:

- ¼ teaspoon ground red pepper or chili powder
- ¼ teaspoon ground turmeric
- ¼ teaspoon salt
- 1 teaspoon honey
- ½ minced clove garlic
- 2 teaspoons whole grain mustard
- 4 pcs 6-oz salmon fillets

Directions:

1. In a small bowl mix well salt, garlic powder, red pepper, turmeric, honey and mustard.
2. Preheat oven to broil and grease a baking dish with cooking spray.
3. Place salmon on baking dish with skin side down and spread evenly mustard mixture on top of salmon.
4. Pop in the oven and broil until flaky around 8 minutes. Serve.

Crisped Coco-Shrimp with Mango Dip

Preparation Time: 10 minutes
Cooking Time: 20 minutes
Servings: 4

Ingredients:

- 1 cup shredded coconut
- 1 lb. raw shrimp, peeled and deveined

- 2 egg whites
- 4 tablespoon tapioca starch
- Pepper and salt to taste

MANGO DIP:

- 1 cup mango, chopped

- 1 jalapeño, thinly minced
- 1 teaspoon lime juice
- 1/3 cup coconut milk
- 3 teaspoon raw honey

Directions:

1. Preheat oven to 400°F. Take a pan with a wire rack on top.
2. In a medium bowl, add tapioca starch and season with pepper and salt.
3. In a second medium bowl, add egg whites and whisk.
4. In a third medium bowl, add coconut.
5. To ready shrimps, dip first in tapioca starch, then egg whites, and then coconut. Place dredged shrimp on wire rack. Repeat until all shrimps are covered. Pop shrimps in the oven and roast for 10 minutes per side.
6. Meanwhile make the dip by adding all ingredients in a blender. Puree until smooth and creamy. Transfer to a dipping bowl. Once shrimps are golden brown, serve with mango dip.

Dill Relish on White Sea Bass

Preparation Time: 10 minutes
Cooking Time: 12 minutes
Servings: 4
Ingredients:

- 1 ½ tablespoon chopped white onion
- 1 ½ teaspoon chopped fresh dill

- 1 lemon, quartered
- 1 teaspoon Dijon mustard
- 1 teaspoon lemon juice
- 1 teaspoon pickled baby capers, drained
- 4 pieces of 4-oz white sea bass fillets

Directions:

1. Preheat oven to 375°F. Prepare four aluminum foil squares and place 1 fillet per foil.
2. Mix lemon juice, mustard, dill, capers and onions in a small bowl. Squeeze a lemon wedge per fish. Divide into 4 the dill spread and drizzle over fillet. Close the foil over the fish securely and pop in the oven. Bake for 12 minutes or until fish is cooked through. Remove from foil and transfer to a serving platter, serve and enjoy.

Dijon Mustard and Lime Marinated Shrimp

Preparation Time: 10 minutes
Cooking Time: 10 minutes
Servings: 8
Ingredients:

- ½ cup fresh lime juice, and lime zest as garnish
- ½ cup rice vinegar
- ½ teaspoon hot sauce

- 1 bay leaf
- 1 cup water
- 1 lb. uncooked shrimp, peeled and deveined
- 1 medium red onion, chopped
- 2 tablespoon capers
- 2 tablespoon Dijon mustard
- 3 garlic cloves

Directions:

1. Mix hot sauce, mustard, capers, lime juice and onion in a shallow baking dish and set aside.
2. Bring to a boil in a large saucepan bay leaf, cloves, vinegar and water. Once boiling, add shrimps and cook for 1 minute stirring continuously. Drain shrimps and pour shrimps into onion mixture.
3. For 1 hour, refrigerate while covered the shrimps.
4. Then serve shrimps cold and garnished with lime zest. Enjoy!

Lean and Green Recipes

Tomatillo and Green Chili Pork Stew

Preparation Time: 10 minutes

Cooking Time: 20 minutes

Servings: 4

Ingredients:

- 2 scallions, chopped
- 2 cloves of garlic
- 1 lb. tomatillos, trimmed and chopped
- 8 large romaine or green lettuce leaves, divided
- 2 serrano chilies, seeds, and membranes
- ½ tsp of dried Mexican oregano (or you can use regular oregano)
- 1 ½ lb. of boneless pork loin, to be cut into bite-sized cubes
- ¼ cup of cilantro, chopped
- ¼ tablespoon (each) salt and paper
- 1 jalapeno, seeds and membranes to be removed and thinly sliced
- 1 cup of sliced radishes
- 4 lime wedges

Directions:

1. Combine scallions, garlic, tomatillos, 4 lettuce leaves, serrano chilies, and oregano in a blender. Then puree until smoot.
2. Put pork and tomatillo mixture in a medium pot; 1-inch of puree should cover the pork; if not, add water until it covers it. Season with pepper and salt, and cover it. Simmer on heat for approximately 20 minutes.
3. Finely shred the remaining lettuce leaves. When the stew is done cooking, garnish with cilantro, radishes, finely shredded lettuce, sliced jalapenos, and lime wedges.

Cloud Bread

Preparation Time: 25 minutes

Cooking Time: 35 minutes

Servings: 3

Ingredients:

- ½ cup of Fat-free 0% Plain Greek Yogurt)
- 3 Eggs, Separated
- 16 teaspoon Cream of Tartar
- 1 Packet sweetener (a granulated sweetener just like stevia)

Directions:

1. Preheat your oven to 300°F. Take a baking dish with a parchment paper.
2. Separate the eggs and put the egg whites in a bowl.
3. In another medium-sized bowl containing the yolks, mix in the sweetener and yogurt.
4. In the bowl containing the egg white, add in the cream of tartar. Beat this mixture until the egg whites turn to stiff peaks. Take the egg yolk mixture and carefully fold it into the egg whites. Be cautious and avoid over-stirring.
5. Scoop out 6 equally-sized "blobs" of the "dough" onto the parchment paper and bake for about 25-35 minutes. (make sure you check when it is 25 minutes, in some ovens, they are done at this timestamp). You will know they are done as they will get brownish at the top and have some crack. Serve!

Avocado Lime Shrimp Salad

Preparation Time: 15 minutes

Cooking Time: 0 minutes

Servings: 2

Ingredients:

- 14 ounces of cooked shrimp, peeled and deveined
- 4 ½ ounces of avocado, diced
- 1 ½ cup of tomato, diced
- ¼ cup of chopped green onion
- ¼ cup of jalapeno diced fine
- 1 teaspoon of olive oil
- 2 tablespoons of lime juice
- 1/8 teaspoon of salt
- 1 tablespoon of chopped cilantro

Directions:

1. Get a small bowl and combine green onion, olive oil, lime juice, pepper, a pinch of salt. Wait for about 5 minutes for all of them to marinate and mellow the flavor of the onion.
2. Get a large bowl and combined chopped shrimp, tomato, avocado, jalapeno. Combine all of the ingredients, add cilantro, and gently toss. Add pepper and salt as desired and serve!

Broccoli Cheddar Breakfast Bake

Preparation Time: 10 minutes

Cooking Time: 45 minutes

Servings: 4

Ingredients:

- 9 eggs
- 6 cups of small broccoli florets
- ¼ teaspoon of salt
- 1 cup of unsweetened almond milk
- ¼ teaspoon of cayenne pepper
- ¼ teaspoon of ground pepper
- Cooking spray
- 4 oz. of shredded, reduced-fat cheddar

Directions:

1. Preheat your oven to about 375°. Take a lightly greased 13 x 9-inch baking dish.
2. In your large microwave-safe, add broccoli and 2 to 3 tablespoons of water.
3. Microwave on high heat for 4 minutes or until it becomes tender. Now transfer the broccoli to a colander to drain excess liquid. Get a medium-sized bowl and whisk the milk, eggs, and seasonings together.
4. Set the broccoli neatly on the bottom of a baking pan. Sprinkle the cheese gently on the broccoli and pour the egg mixture on top of it. Bake for about 45 minutes or until the center is set and the top forms a light brown crust.

Grilled Mahi Mahi with Jicama Slaw

Preparation Time: 20 minutes

Cooking Time: 10 minutes

Servings: 4

Ingredients:

- 1 teaspoon each for pepper and salt, divided
- 1 tablespoon of lime juice, divided
- 4 tablespoon of extra virgin olive oil
- 4 raw mahi-mahi fillets
- ½ cucumber, thinly cutted
- 1 jicama, thinly cutted
- 1 cup of alfalfa sprouts
- 2 cups of coarsely chopped

Directions:

1. Combine ½ teaspoon of both pepper and salt, 1 teaspoon of lime juice, and 2 teaspoons of oil in a small bowl. Then brush the mahi-mahi fillets all through with the olive oil mixture.
2. Grill the mahi-mahi on medium-high heat until it becomes done in about 5 minutes, turn it to the other side, and let it be done for about 5 minutes. (You will have an internal temperature of about 145°F).
3. For the slaw, combine the watercress, cucumber, jicama, and alfalfa sprouts in a bowl. Now combine ½ teaspoon of both pepper and salt, 2 teaspoons of lime juice, and 2 tablespoons of extra virgin oil in a small bowl. Drizzle it over slaw and toss together to combine.

Rosemary Cauliflower Rolls

Preparation Time: 10 minutes

Cooking Time: 30 minutes

Servings: 3

Ingredients:

- 1/3 cup of almond flour
- 4 cups of riced cauliflower
- 1/3 cup of reduced-fat, shredded mozzarella
- 2 eggs
- 2 tablespoons of fresh rosemary, finely chopped
- ½ teaspoon of salt

Directions:

1. Preheat your oven to 400°F. Take a lightly greased and foil-lined baking sheet.
2. Combine all the listed ingredients in a medium-sized bowl
3. Scoop cauliflower mixture into 12 evenly sized rolls/biscuits onto the baking pan. Bake until it turns golden brown, about 30 minutes. Serve warm!

Note: if you want to have the outside of the rolls/biscuits crisp, then broil for some minutes before serving.

Mediterranean Chicken Salad

Preparation Time: 5 minutes
Cooking Time: 25 minutes
Servings: 4
Ingredients:
FOR CHICKEN:

- 1 ¾ lb. boneless, skinless chicken breast
- ¼ teaspoon of pepper and salt
- 1 ½ tablespoon of butter, melted

FOR MEDITERRANEAN SALAD:

- 1 cup of sliced cucumber
- 6 cups of romaine lettuce, chopped
- 10 pitted Kalamata olives
- 1 pint of cherry tomatoes
- 1/3 cup of reduced-fat feta cheese
- ¼ teaspoon of pepper and salt
- 2 tablespoons of lemon juice

Directions:
1. Preheat your oven or grill to about 350°F. Take a lightly greased and foil-lined baking sheet.
2. Season the chicken with salt, butter, and black pepper.
3. Roast or grill chicken for 25 minutes. Once your chicken breasts are cooked, remove and keep aside to rest for 5 minutes. Combine all the salad ingredients you have and toss everything together very well. Serve!

Lemon Garlic Oregano Chicken with Asparagus

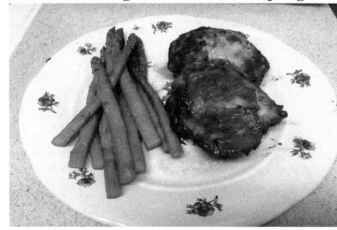

Preparation Time: 5 minutes
Cooking Time: 40 minutes
Servings: 4
Ingredients:

- 1 small lemon, juiced (this should be about 2 tablespoons of lemon juice)
- 1 ¾ lb. of bone-in, skinless chicken thighs
- 2 tablespoons of fresh oregano, minced
- 2 cloves of garlic, minced
- 2 lbs. of asparagus, trimmed
- ¼ teaspoon each or less for black pepper and salt

Directions:
1. Preheat the oven to about 350°F. Take a lightly greased and foil-lined baking sheet.
2. Put the chicken in a medium-sized bowl. Add the garlic, oregano, lemon juice, pepper, and salt and toss together to combine. Roast the chicken in the oven for 40 minutes. Once the chicken thighs have been cooked, remove and keep aside to rest.
3. Steam the asparagus on a stovetop or in a microwave to the desired doneness.
4. Serve asparagus with the roasted chicken thighs. Serve!

Sheet Pan Chicken Fajita Lettuce Wraps

Preparation Time: 15 minutes

Cooking Time: 30 minutes

Servings: 2

Ingredients:

- 1 lb. chicken breast, thinly sliced into strips
- 2 teaspoon of olive oil
- 2 bell peppers, thinly sliced into strips
- 2 teaspoon of fajita seasoning
- 6 leaves from a romaine heart
- Juice of half a lime
- ¼ cup plain of non-fat Greek yogurt

Directions:

1. Preheat your oven to about 400°F. Take a lightly greased and foil-lined baking sheet.
2. Combine all of the ingredients except for lettuce in a large plastic bag that can be resealed. Mix very well to coat vegetables and chicken with oil and seasoning evenly.
3. Spread the contents of the bag evenly on a foil-lined baking sheet. Bake it for about2 5-30 minutes.
4. Serve on lettuce leaves and topped with Greek yogurt.

Savory Cilantro Salmon

Preparation Time: 1 hour 10 minutes

Cooking Time: 30 minutes

Servings: 4

Ingredients:

- 2 tablespoons of fresh lime or lemon
- 4 cups of fresh cilantro, divided
- 2 tablespoon of hot red pepper sauce
- ½ teaspoon of salt. Divided
- 1 teaspoon of cumin
- 4, 7 oz. of salmon filets
- ½ cup of (4 oz.) water
- 2 cups of sliced red bell pepper
- 2 cups of sliced yellow bell pepper
- 2 cups of sliced green bell pepper
- Olive oil to grease
- ½ teaspoon of pepper

Directions:

1. Get a blender or food processor and combine half of the cilantro, lime juice or lemon, cumin, hot red pepper sauce, water, and salt; then puree until they become smooth. Transfer the marinade gotten into a large re-sealable plastic bag.
2. Add salmon to marinade. Seal the bag, squeeze out air that might have been trapped inside, turn to coat salmon. Refrigerate for about 1 hour.
3. After marinating, preheat your oven to about 400°F. Arrange the pepper slices in a single layer in a slightly greased, medium-sized baking dish. Bake it for 20 minutes, turn the pepper slices once.
4. Drain your salmon and do away with the marinade. Crust the upper part of the salmon with the remaining chopped, fresh cilantro. Place salmon on the top of the pepper slices and bake for about 12-14 minutes until you observe that the fish flakes easily when it is being tested with a fork. Enjoy!

Salmon Florentine

Preparation Time: 5 minutes

Cooking Time: 30 minutes

Servings: 4

Ingredients:

- 1 ½ cups of chopped cherry tomatoes
- ½ cup of chopped green onions
- 2 garlic cloves, minced
- 1 teaspoon of olive oil
- 1 quantity of 12 oz. package frozen chopped spinach, thawed and patted dry
- ¼ teaspoon of crushed red pepper flakes
- ½ cup of part-skim ricotta cheese
- ¼ teaspoon each for pepper and salt
- 4 quantities of 5 ½ oz. wild salmon fillets
- Cooking spray

Directions:

1. Preheat the oven to 350°F. Take a lightly greased and foil-lined baking sheet.

2. Get a medium skillet to cook onions in oil until they start to soften, which should be in about 2 minutes. You can then add garlic inside the skillet and cook for an extra 1 minute. Add the spinach, red pepper flakes, tomatoes, pepper, and salt. Cook for 2 minutes while stirring. Remove the pan from the heat and let it cool for about 10 minutes. Stir in the ricotta

3. Put a quarter of the spinach mixture on top of each salmon fillet. Place the fillets on baking pan and bake it for 15 minutes or until you are sure that the salmon has been thoroughly cooked. Serve.

Tomato Braised Cauliflower with Chicken

Preparation Time: 10 minutes
Cooking Time: 30 minutes
Servings: 4
Ingredients:

- 4 garlic cloves, sliced
- 3 scallions, to be trimmed and cut into 1-inch pieces
- ¼ teaspoon of dried oregano
- ¼ teaspoon of crushed red pepper flakes
- 4 ½ cups of cauliflower
- 1 ½ cups of diced canned tomatoes
- 1 cup of fresh basil, gently torn
- ½ teaspoon each of pepper and salt, divided
- 1 ½ teaspoon of olive oil
- 1 ½ lb. of boneless, skinless chicken breasts

Directions:

1. Get a saucepan and combine the garlic, scallions, oregano, crushed red pepper, cauliflower, and tomato, and add ¼ cup of water. Get everything boil together and add ¼ teaspoon of pepper and salt for seasoning, then cover the pot with a lid. Let it simmer for 10 minutes and stir as often as possible until you observe that the cauliflower is tender. Now, wrap up the seasoning with the remaining ¼ teaspoon of pepper and salt.

2. Toss the chicken breast with olive oil olive and let it roast in the oven to 450°F for 20 minutes. Let the chicken rest for 10 minutes. Slice the chicken and serve on a bed of tomato braised cauliflower.

Cheeseburger Soup

Preparation Time: 20 minutes
Cooking Time: 25 minutes
Servings: 4
Ingredients:

- ¼ cup of chopped onion
- 1 quantity of 14.5 oz. diced tomato
- 1 lb. of 90% lean ground beef
- ¾ cup of diced celery
- 2 teaspoon of Worcestershire sauce
- 3 cups of low sodium chicken broth
- ¼ teaspoon of salt
- 1 teaspoon of dried parsley
- 7 cups of baby spinach
- ¼ teaspoon of ground pepper
- 4 oz. of reduced-fat shredded cheddar cheese

Directions:

1. Get a large pot and cook the beef for 15 minutes. Add the celery, onion, and sauté until it becomes tender. Remove from the fire and drain excess liquid. Stir in the broth, tomatoes, parsley, Worcestershire sauce, pepper, and salt. Cover and allow it to simmer on low heat for about 20 minutes.

2. Add spinach and leave it to cook until it becomes wilted in about 1-3 minutes. Top each of your servings with 1 ounce of cheese. Serve warm.

Braised Collard Greens in Peanut Sauce with Pork Tenderloin

Preparation Time: 20 minutes   **Cooking Time:** 1 hour 12 minutes   **Servings:** 4
Ingredients:

- 2 cups of chicken stock
- 12 cups of chopped collard greens
- 5 tablespoon of powdered peanut butter
- 3 cloves of garlic, crushed

- 1 teaspoon of salt
- ½ teaspoon of allspice
- ½ teaspoon of black pepper
- 2 teaspoon of lemon juice
- ¾ teaspoon of hot sauce
- 1 ½ lb. of pork tenderloin

Directions:

1. Get a pot with a tight-fitting lid and combine the collards with the garlic, chicken stock, hot sauce, and half of the pepper and salt. Cook on low heat for about 1 hour or until the collards become tender.
2. Once the collards are tender, stir in the allspice, lemon juice. And powdered peanut butter. Keep warm.
3. Season the pork tenderloin with the remaining pepper and salt, and broil in a toaster oven for 10 minutes when you have an internal temperature of 145°F. Make sure to turn the tenderloin every 2 minutes to achieve an even browning all over. After that, you can take away the pork from the oven and allow it to rest for like 5 minutes.
4. Slice the pork as you will and serve.

Delicious Recipes

Parmesan Zucchini Rounds

Preparation Time: 25 minutes

Cooking Time: 20 minutes

Servings: 4

Ingredients:

- 4 zucchinis; sliced
- 1 ½ cups parmesan; grated
- ¼ cup parsley; chopped.
- 1 egg; whisked
- 1 egg white; whisked
- ½ tsp. garlic powder
- Cooking spray

Directions:

1. Take a bowl and mix the egg with egg whites, parmesan, parsley and garlic powder and whisk.
2. Dredge each zucchini slice in this mix, place them all in your air fryer's basket, grease them with cooking spray and cook at 370°F for 20 minutes. Divide between plates and serve as a side dish.

Green Bean Casserole

Preparation Time: 25 minutes

Cooking Time: 20 minutes

Servings: 4

Ingredients:

- 1 lb. fresh green beans, edges trimmed
- ½ oz. pork rinds, finely ground
- 1 oz. full-fat cream cheese
- ½ cup heavy whipping cream.
- ¼ cup diced yellow onion
- ½ cup chopped white mushrooms
- ½ cup chicken broth
- 4 tbsp. unsalted butter.
- ¼ tsp. xanthan gum

Directions:

1. Overheat melt the butter in a skillet, then sauté the onion and mushrooms until soft, about 3-5 minutes.
2. Add the heavy cream, cream cheese, and broth to the skillet. Lightly beat until smooth. Boil and then simmer. Put the xanthan gum in the pan and remove from heat.
3. Cut green beans into 2-inch pieces and place in 4-cup round pan. Pour sauce mixture over them and stir until covered. Fill the plate with ground pork rinds. Place in the fryer basket at 320°F for 15 minutes.
4. The top will be a golden and green bean fork when fully cooked. Serve hot.

Excellent Warrior Omelet

Preparation Time: 5 minutes

Cooking Time: 10 minutes

Servings: 1 to 2

Ingredients:

- ½ teaspoon olive oil
- ½ avocado sliced
- 2 ½ green onions, diced
- 2 organic small tomatoes
- 1 cup spinach leaves
- 2 large eggs, scrambled

Directions:

1. Heat olive oil on low in nonstick omelet pan. Saute onions until tender. Add eggs and cook properly on low for about 3 minutes, then add quickly the remaining ingredients, chopped.
2. Finally, fold and flip omelet until eggs are fully cooked. Serve warm.

Legendary Omelet with Avocado and Pico De Gallo

Preparation Time: 15 minutes   **Cooking Time:** 10 minutes   **Servings:** 2

Ingredients:

- 2 tablespoons Pico de Gallo
- Egg – 1 large
- Egg white – 1 large

- Avocado – 1 sliced
- Salt and pepper to taste
- 2 tablespoons Olive oil

Directions:
1. In a small or maybe medium bowl, please beat the egg white and egg; then season with salt and pepper.
2. Heat olive oil on medium in a nonstick skillet. Pour the eggs and cook for 3 minutes, or until set.
3. Transfer to a plate, top with Pico de Gallo and avocado and enjoy.

Awesome Spiced Orange Glazed Ham

Preparation Time: 40 minutes   **Cooking Time:** 2 hours 10 minutes   **Servings:** 2
Ingredients:
- 1 ready-to-eat, cooked ham, bone-in, shank end or maybe butt end, around 9-10 pounds (or heavier, if you may prefer)
- About 2 to 3 tablespoons maple syrup

FOR THE RUB:
- About 1 or 2 teaspoons onion powder
- About 1/2 teaspoon cayenne
- 1/2 teaspoon smoked paprika
- 1/2 teaspoon cinnamon
- 1/2 teaspoon ground cloves
- About 1.5 teaspoon garlic powder
- FOR GARNISH:
- 4 navel oranges, cut in half

FOR THE GLAZE:
- 1/2 cup coconut aminos
- 1 teaspoon chili powder
- About 2.5 tablespoons maple syrup
- 1/2 teaspoon smoked paprika
- About 1/2 teaspoon fish sauce
- 2 cups orange juice
- Zest of about 1/2 an orange

Directions:
1. Preheat oven to 320 °F.
2. Combine onion powder, garlic powder, smoked paprika, ground clove, cinnamon, and cayenne.
3. Put the ham into a pan and cover with the maple syrup. Rub the spice mixture onto the ham, completely covering it and letting it get between the slices. Cover the ham with foil, put into the oven and bake for about 1.5 hours.
4. Then half an hour before the ham is done, add orange juice, coconut aminos, orange zest, maple syrup, fish sauce, smoked paprika and chili powder into a large pan and mix well.
5. Cook over medium heat for about 35 minutes, stirring frequently. When it is reduced by 1/3 and begins to boil, remove from heat. Remove foil from the ham, when done, and glaze the entire ham with half of the prepare orange glaze. Stick a few toothpicks through the ham to prevent unfolding and put orange halve around.
6. Next, put the ham back into the oven and cook properly for about 30 to 35 more minutes at 400°F.
7. Remove and glaze with the rest of the orange glaze. Finally serve.

Quick Eggs Benedict on Artichoke Hearts

Preparation Time: 20 minutes
Cooking Time: 1 hours 10 minutes
Servings: 2
Ingredients:
- Salt and pepper to taste (optional)
- 3 turkey breasts, finely chopped
- ½ cup balsamic vinegar
- About 2.5 artichoke hearts
- 2 eggs
- Hollandaise sauce
- About 1 cup melted ghee
- 3 egg yolks
- Pinch of paprika
- ¾ tablespoon lemon juice
- Pinch of salt
- 1 egg white

Directions: Line baking sheet with foil and preheat oven to 370° F.
1. Remove artichoke hearts from their dressing and place them in the balsamic vinegar for at least 15 to 20 minutes.
2. Fill a pot of water and simmer it on your stove for the Hollandaise sauce.

3. Melt the ghee in a separate saucepan.
4. Separate your eggs, placing the yolks in a cooking bowl and hang on to the egg whites.
5. Take the artichoke hearts out of the marinade and then place them on the baking pan. Brush them with the egg white before placing the turkey breasts over the artichokes' tops. Put in the oven for 25 minutes.
6. Whisk the egg yolks in the lemon juice, then place the bowl (preferably stainless steel) over the pot of simmering water. This should create a double boiler. Then, slowly add the ghee and a little bit of salt. Whisk it until it doubles in size and looks silky, then set aside. Turn up the heat on the pot of water and get it boiling.
7. Crack the eggs in one at a time into a ladle, and then slide that spoon full of egg into the water. This will poach the eggs that go on top of the turkey breasts. Let them sit in the water for 2 minutes, and then remove.
8. Take out the artichoke hearts and turkey breasts (if not already out) and lay them on a plate.
9. Finally place the poached egg on top and pour the Hollandaise sauce on top.
10. Sprinkle with salt, pepper, and paprika to taste. Enjoy!

Wonderful Paleo Crock Pot Chicken Soup

Preparation Time: 40 minutes
Cooking Time: 6 hours 10 minutes
Servings: 5
Ingredients:

- 4 cups filtered water
- 3 carrots, diced
- 3 celery stalks, diced
- About 1 teaspoon fresh ground pepper
- 1 Tablespoon herbs de Provence
- 2 chicken thighs, organic, with bone, with skin
- 1 teaspoon sea salt
- 2 chicken breasts, organic, with bone, with skin
- About 1.5 teaspoon apple cider vinegar
- 1 medium onion, diced

Directions:
1. Place all the ingredients in a pot ensuring the chicken is placed on top of the vegetables, bone should be side down. Add 4 cups of water, to cover the ingredients and cook on low for about 5 to 6 hours, until meat flakes off bone and vegetables are fork tender. Once cooked, take out the chicken. Remove skin and bones.
2. Shred the chicken with 2 forks.
3. Return pieces to the soup. Stir well. Taste. Season if needed. Finally serve in bowls.

Rich Omelet Under Applesauce

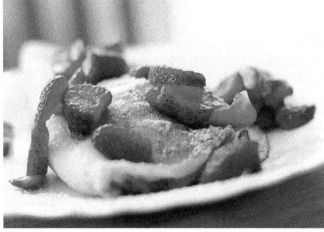

Preparation Time: 15 minutes
Cooking Time: 30 minutes
Servings: 1 dozen truffles
Ingredients:

- About 1/2 teaspoon dash vanilla
- 2-3 strawberries, sliced
- About 1/2 teaspoon dash cinnamon
- 1/2 apple or 2 tablespoons applesauce
- 3-4 eggs

Directions:
1. Pre-heat the skillet over medium heat.
2. Break the eggs into the bowl, add cinnamon and vanilla, stir thoroughly
3. Then pour the mixture on the skillet, cook it properly for about 2 to 5 minutes till it mostly ready, toss it.
4. Cook it properly for about 2 minutes, transfer it on the plate.
5. Finally distribute the applesauce over the half of the omelet, add strawberry slices, fold it with another half and cut into 2 portions. Serve!

Delicious Zucchini Smoothie

Preparation Time: 10 Minutes
Cooking Time: 15 minutes

Servings: 3

Ingredients:

- 1 Brown Onion, chopped
- 2 Cups of water
- 2 ½ tbsps. Coconut Oil
- 1 Large Zucchini, sliced

Directions:

1. Heat the coconut oil in a pan on low and fry the onions until golden brown. Add the Zucchini and cook properly under medium heat until tender. Add 2 cups of water and boil. When boiling blend together.
2. Finally add a dash of salt to taste. Enjoy!

Yummy Kale Omelets

Preparation Time: 5 minutes

Cooking Time: 10 minutes

Servings: 2

Ingredients:

- Salt and pepper
- 1 cup chopped Kale
- 1 ½ tablespoons fresh chives
- Eggs – 3
- Butter – 1 tablespoon

Directions:

1. First of all, place a frying pan over medium heat then add butter and heat. Add kale to the pan then cook properly for about 5 to 10 minutes or until soft. Beat the eggs in a bowl then add fresh chives, pepper and salt.
2. Add egg mixture to the frying pan then swirl the pan for the mixture to spread to the edges.
3. Cook properly on low heat until well set at the top. Finally fold over and serve.

Unique Banana Pancakes

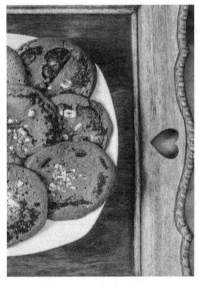

Preparation Time: 5 to 10 Minutes

Cooking Time: 15 minutes

Servings: 2 to 4

Ingredients:

- Vanilla Extract, dash (Optional)
- 1 free-range egg
- About 1.5 tsp cinnamon
- 1 tsp of coconut (Shredded)
- 1 banana (Mashed)
- Seeds for garnish (Optional)

Directions:

1. First of all, mash one whole banana and lightly beat with an egg.
2. For extra flavor, add coconut chips, vanilla extract (just a dash) and cinnamon.
3. Put this in a pan with a bit of oil on the bottom (or pour this mixture into a frying pan, if you have) and cook properly as you would a regular pancake.
4. Serve with garnish. Enjoy!

Iconic Italian Pulled Pork Ragu

Preparation Time: 10 Minutes

Cooking Time: 2 hours 30 minutes

Servings: 4

Ingredients:

- 1 ½ tablespoon parsley, divided
- Salt and pepper, to taste
- 2 bay leaves
- 1 teaspoon olive oil
- 4 garlic cloves, minced
- 2 ½ sprigs fresh thyme
- 4 cups chopped tomatoes
- 1 small jar roasted red peppers, drained
- 18 ounces pork tenderloin

Directions:

1. Sprinkle the pork tenderloin with salt and pepper. Smash garlic cloves with a knife. Finely chop tomatoes.

2. Add oil to a preheated large pot. Add garlic and sauté over medium-high heat for about 2 minutes, until golden; then remove the garlic with a slotted spoon and set aside. Add pork and brown it on each side for 3 minutes.
3. Add tomatoes, fresh thyme, red peppers, bay leave and half of the chopped parsley.
4. Bring to a boil, cover, and cook properly on low heat for about 2.5 hours, until the fork is fork tender.
5. Remove bay leaves and then shred the pork with 2 forks; serve over pasta topped with the remaining parsley.

Hummus with Ground Lamb

Preparation Time: 10 minutes
Cooking Time: 15 minutes
Servings: 8
Ingredients:

- 10 ounces hummus
- 12 ounces lamb meat, ground
- ½ cup pomegranate seeds
- ¼ cup parsley, chopped
- 1 tablespoon olive oil
- Pita chips for serving

Directions:
1. Heat oil in a pan over medium-high heat, add the meat, and brown for 15 minutes stirring often.
2. Spread the hummus on a platter, spread the ground lamb all over, also spread the pomegranate seeds and the parsley and serve with pita chips as a snack.

Bulgur Lamb Meatballs

Preparation Time: 10 minutes
Cooking Time: 15 minutes
Servings: 6
Ingredients:

- 1 and ½ cups Greek yogurt
- ½ teaspoon cumin, ground
- 1 cup cucumber, shredded
- ½ teaspoon garlic, minced
- A pinch of salt and black pepper
- 1 cup bulgur
- 2 cups water
- 1-pound lamb, ground
- ¼ cup parsley, chopped
- ¼ cup shallots, chopped
- ½ teaspoon allspice, ground
- ½ teaspoon cinnamon powder
- 1 tablespoon olive oil

Directions:
1. Combine the bulgur with the water in a bowl, cover the bowl, leave aside for 10 minutes, drain and transfer to a bowl. Add the meat, the yogurt and the rest of the ingredients except the oil, stir well and shape medium meatballs out of this mix.
2. Heat oil in a pan over medium-high heat, add the meatballs, cook them for 7 minutes on each side, arrange them all on a platter and serve as an appetizer.

Wrapped Plums

Preparation Time: 5 minutes
Cooking Time: 0 minutes
Servings: 8
Ingredients:

- 2 ounces prosciutto, cut into 16 pieces
- 4 plums, quartered
- 1 tablespoon chives, chopped
- A pinch of red pepper flakes, crushed

Directions:
1. Wrap each plum quarter in a prosciutto slice.
2. Arrange them all on a platter, sprinkle the chives and pepper flakes all over and serve.

White Bean Dip

Preparation Time: 10 minutes
Cooking Time: 0 minute

Servings: 4
Ingredients:

- 15 ounces canned white beans, drained
- 6 cups canned artichoke hearts, drained, chopped
- 4 garlic cloves, minced
- 1 tablespoon basil, chopped
- 2 tablespoons olive oil
- Juice of ½ lemon
- Zest of ½ lemon, grated
- Salt and black pepper to taste

Directions:
1. In your food processor, combine the beans with the artichokes and the rest of the ingredients except the oil and pulse well.
2. Add the oil gradually, pulse the mix again, divide into cups and serve as a party dip.

Eggplant Dip

Preparation Time: 10 minutes
Cooking Time: 40 minutes

Servings: 4
Ingredients:

- 1 eggplant, poked with a fork
- 2 tablespoons tahini paste
- 2 tablespoons lemon juice
- 2 garlic cloves, minced
- 1 tablespoon olive oil
- Salt and black pepper to the taste
- 1 tablespoon parsley, chopped

Directions:
1. Put the eggplant in a roasting pan, bake at 400° F for 40 minutes, cool down, peel and transfer to your food processor.
2. Add the rest of the remaining ingredients except the parsley, pulse well, divide into small bowls and serve as an appetizer with the parsley sprinkled on top.

Cucumber Bites

Preparation Time: 10 minutes
Cooking Time: 0 minutes
Servings: 12
Ingredients:

- 1 English cucumber, sliced into 32 rounds
- 10 ounces hummus
- 16 cherry tomatoes, halved
- 1 tablespoon parsley, chopped
- 1-ounce feta cheese, crumbled

Directions:
1. Spread the hummus on each cucumber round,
2. divide the tomato halves on each, sprinkle the cheese and parsley on to and serve as an appetizer.

Stuffed Avocado

Preparation Time: 10 minutes
Cooking Time: 0 minute
Servings: 2
Ingredients:

- 1 avocado, halved and pitted
- 10 ounces canned tuna, drained
- 2 tablespoons sun-dried tomatoes, chopped
- 1 and ½ tablespoon basil pesto
- 2 tablespoons black olives, pitted and chopped
- Salt and black pepper to the taste
- 2 teaspoons pine nuts, toasted and chopped
- 1 tablespoon basil, chopped

Directions:
1. Combine the tuna with the sun-dried tomatoes in a bowl, and the rest of the ingredients except the avocado and stir. Stuff the avocado halves with the tuna mix and serve as an appetizer.

Goat Cheese and Chives Spread

Preparation Time: 10 minutes
Cooking Time: 0 minute
Servings: 4
Ingredients:

- 2 ounces goat cheese, crumbled
- ¾ cup sour cream
- 2 tablespoons chives, chopped
- 1 tablespoon lemon juice
- Salt and black pepper to the taste
- 2 tablespoons extra virgin olive oil

Directions:

1. Mix the goat cheese with the cream and the rest of the ingredients in a bowl and whisk really well.
2. Keep in the fridge for 10 minutes and serve as a party spread.

Cucumber Sandwich Bites

Preparation Time: 5 minutes   **Cooking Time:** 0 minutes   **Servings:** 12
Ingredients:

- 1 cucumber, sliced
- 8 slices whole wheat bread
- 2 tablespoons cream cheese, soft
- 1 tablespoon chives, chopped
- ¼ cup avocado, peeled, and mashed
- 1 teaspoon mustard
- Salt and black pepper to taste

Directions:

1. Spread the mashed avocado on each bread slice, also spread the rest of the ingredients except the cucumber slices.
2. Divide the cucumber slices on the bread slices, cut each slice in thirds, arrange on a plate. Serve as an appetizer.

Creamy Spinach and Shallots Dip

Preparation Time: 10 minutes
Cooking Time: 0 minutes
Servings: 4
Ingredients:

- 1-pound spinach, roughly chopped
- 2 shallots, chopped
- 2 tablespoons mint, chopped
- ¾ cup cream cheese, soft
- Salt and black pepper to the taste

Directions:

1. Combine the spinach with the shallots and the rest of the ingredients in a blender, and pulse well.
2. Divide into small bowls and serve as a party dip.

Cucumber Rolls

Preparation Time: 5 minutes
Cooking Time: 0 minutes
Servings: 6
Ingredients:

- 1 big cucumber, sliced lengthwise
- 1 tablespoon parsley, chopped
- 8 ounces canned tuna, drained and mashed
- Salt and black pepper to the taste
- 1 teaspoon lime juice

Directions:

1. Arrange cucumber slices on a working surface, divide the rest of the ingredients, and roll.
2. Arrange all the rolls on a surface and serve as an appetizer.

Tomato Salsa

Preparation Time: 5 minutes
Cooking Time: 0 minutes
Servings: 6
Ingredients:

- 1 garlic clove, minced
- 4 tablespoons olive oil
- 5 tomatoes, cubed
- 1 tablespoon balsamic vinegar
- ¼ cup basil, chopped

- 1 tablespoon parsley, chopped
- 1 tablespoon chives, chopped
- Salt and black pepper to the taste
- Pita chips for serving

Directions:
1. Mix the tomatoes with the garlic in a bowl, and the rest of the ingredients except the pita chips and stir.
2. Divide into small cups and serve with the pita chips on the side.

Avocado Dip

Preparation Time: 5 minutes

Cooking Time: 0 minutes

Servings: 8

Ingredients:
- ½ cup heavy cream
- 1 green chili pepper, chopped
- Salt and pepper to taste
- 4 avocados, peeled and chopped
- 1 cup cilantro, chopped
- ¼ cup lime juice

Directions:
1. Pour the cream with the avocados and the rest of the ingredients in a blender and pulse well.
2. Divide the mix into bowls and serve cold as a party dip.

Chili Mango and Watermelon Salsa

Preparation Time: 5 minutes

Cooking Time: 0 minutes

Servings: 12

Ingredients:
- 1 red tomato, chopped
- Salt and black pepper to the taste
- 1 cup watermelon, seedless, cubed
- 1 red onion, chopped
- 2 mangos, peeled and chopped
- 2 chili peppers, chopped
- ¼ cup cilantro, chopped
- 3 tablespoons lime juice
- Pita chips for serving

Directions:
1. In a bowl, mix the tomato with the peeled watermelon, the onion and the rest of the ingredients except the pita chips and toss well. Divide the mix into small cups and serve with pita chips on the side.

Feta Artichoke Dip

Preparation Time: 10 minutes

Cooking Time: 30 minutes

Servings: 8

Ingredients:
- 8 ounces artichoke hearts, drained
- ¾ cup basil, chopped
- ¾ cup green olives, pitted and chopped
- 1 cup parmesan cheese, grated
- 5 ounces feta cheese, crumbled

Directions:
1. In your food processor, mix the chopped artichokes with the basil and the rest of the ingredients, pulse well, and transfer to a baking dish.
2. Place in the oven, bake at 375° F for 30 minutes. Serve as a party dip.

Dessert

Chocolate Bars

Preparation Time: 10 minutes
Cooking Time: 20 minutes
Servings: 16
Ingredients:

- 15 oz cream cheese, softened
- 15 oz unsweetened dark chocolate
- 1 tsp vanilla
- 10 drops liquid stevia

Directions:

1. Grease 8-inch square dish and set aside.
2. In a saucepan dissolve chocolate over low heat. Add stevia and vanilla and stir well. Remove pan from heat and set aside.
3. Add cream cheese into the blender and blend until smooth. Add melted chocolate mixture into the cream cheese and blend until just combined. Transfer mixture into the prepared dish and spread evenly and place in the refrigerator until firm. Slice and serve.

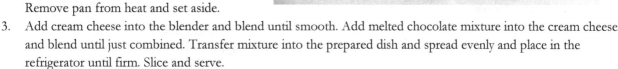

Blueberry Muffins

Preparation Time: 15 minutes
Cooking Time: 35 minutes
Servings: 12
Ingredients:

- 2 eggs
- 1/2 cup fresh blueberries
- 1 cup heavy cream
- 2 cups almond flour
- 1/4 tsp lemon zest
- 1/2 tsp lemon extract
- 1 tsp baking powder
- 5 drops stevia
- 1/4 cup butter, melted

Directions:

1. Heat the cooker to 350° F. Line muffin tin with cupcake liners and set aside.
2. Add eggs into the bowl and whisk until mix.
3. Add remaining ingredients and mix to combine.
4. Pour mixture into the prepared muffin tin and bake for 25 minutes.
5. Serve and enjoy.

Chia Pudding

Preparation Time: 20 minutes
Cooking Time: 0 minutes
Servings: 2
Ingredients:

- 4 tbsp chia seeds

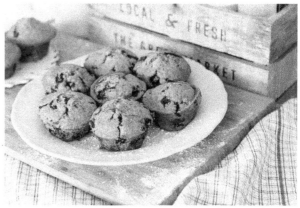

- 1 cup unsweetened coconut milk
- 1/2 cup raspberries

Directions:

1. Add raspberry and coconut milk into a blender and blend until smooth. Pour mixture into the glass jar.
2. Add chia seeds in a jar and stir well. Seal the jar with a lid and shake well and place in the refrigerator for 3 hours.
3. Serve chilled and enjoy.

Avocado Pudding

Preparation Time: 20 minutes

Cooking Time: 0 minutes

Servings: 8

Ingredients:

- 2 ripe avocados, pitted and cut into pieces
- 1 tbsp fresh lime juice
- 14 oz can coconut milk
- 2 tsp liquid stevia
- 2 tsp vanilla

Directions:

1. Inside the blender add all ingredients and blend until smooth.
2. Serve immediately and enjoy.

Peanut Butter Coconut Popsicle

Preparation Time: 15 minutes

Cooking Time: 0 minutes

Servings: 12

Ingredients:

- 1/2 cup peanut butter
- 1 tsp liquid stevia
- 2 cans unsweetened coconut milk

Directions:

1. In the blender add all the listed ingredients and blend until smooth.
2. Pour mixture into the Popsicle molds and place in the freezer for 4 hours or until set.
3. Serve and enjoy.

Delicious Brownie Bites

Preparation Time: 30 minutes

Cooking Time: 0 minutes

Servings: 13

Ingredients:

- 1/4 cup unsweetened chocolate chips
- 1/4 cup unsweetened cocoa powder
- 1 cup pecans, chopped
- 1/2 cup almond butter
- 1/2 tsp vanilla
- 1/4 cup monk fruit sweetener
- 1/8 tsp pink salt

Directions:

1. Add pecans, sweetener, vanilla, almond butter, cocoa powder, and salt into the food processor and process until well combined. Transfer brownie mixture into the large bowl. Add chocolate chips and fold well.
2. Make small round shape balls from brownie mixture and place onto a baking tray.
3. Place in the freezer for 20 minutes. Serve and enjoy.

Pumpkin Balls

Preparation Time: 1 hour 15 minutes

Cooking Time: 0 minutes

Servings: 18

Ingredients:

- 1 cup almond butter
- 5 drops liquid stevia
- 2 tbsp coconut flour
- 2 tbsp pumpkin puree
- 1 tsp pumpkin pie spice

Directions: Mix together pumpkin puree in a large bowl, and almond butter until well combined.

1. Add liquid stevia, pumpkin pie spice, and coconut flour and mix well.
2. Make small balls from mixture and place onto a baking tray.
3. Place in the freezer for 1 hour. Serve and enjoy.

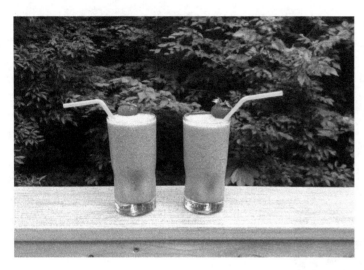

Smooth Peanut Butter Cream

Preparation Time: 10 minutes
Cooking Time: 0 minutes
Servings: 8
Ingredients:

- 1/4 cup peanut butter
- 4 overripe bananas, chopped
- 1/3 cup cocoa powder
- 1/4 tsp vanilla extract
- 1/8 tsp salt

Directions:

1. In the blender add all the listed ingredients and blend until smooth.
2. Serve immediately and enjoy.

Vanilla Avocado Popsicles

Preparation Time: 20 minutes
Cooking Time: 0 minutes
Servings: 6
Ingredients:

- 2 avocadoes
- 1 tsp vanilla
- 1 cup almond milk
- 1 tsp liquid stevia
- 1/2 cup unsweetened cocoa powder

Directions:

1. In the blender add all the listed ingredients and blend smoothly. Pour blended mixture into the Popsicle molds and place in the freezer until set. Serve and enjoy.

Chocolate Popsicle

Preparation Time: 20 minutes
Cooking Time: 10 minutes
Servings: 6
Ingredients:

- 4 oz unsweetened chocolate, chopped
- 6 drops liquid stevia
- 1 1/2 cups heavy cream

Directions:

1. Add heavy cream into the microwave-safe bowl and microwave until just begins the boiling. Add chocolate into the heavy cream and set aside for 5 minutes. Add liquid stevia into the heavy cream mixture and stir until chocolate is melted. Pour mixture into the Popsicle molds and place in freezer for 4 hours or until set.
2. Serve and enjoy.

Raspberry Ice Cream

Preparation Time: 10 minutes   **Cooking Time:** 0 minutes   **Servings:** 2
Ingredients:

- 1 cup frozen raspberries
- 1/2 cup heavy cream
- 1/8 tsp stevia powder

Directions:
1. Blend all the listed ingredients in a blender until smooth.
2. Serve immediately and enjoy.

Chocolate Frosty

Preparation Time: 20 minutes
Cooking Time: 0 minutes
Servings: 4
Ingredients:
- 2 tbsp unsweetened cocoa powder
- 1 cup heavy whipping cream
- 1 tbsp almond butter
- 5 drops liquid stevia
- 1 tsp vanilla

Directions:
1. Add cream into the medium bowl and beat using the hand mixer for 5 minutes. Add remaining ingredients and blend until thick cream form. Pour in serving bowls and place them in the freezer for 30 minutes.
2. Serve and enjoy.

Chocolate Almond Butter Brownie

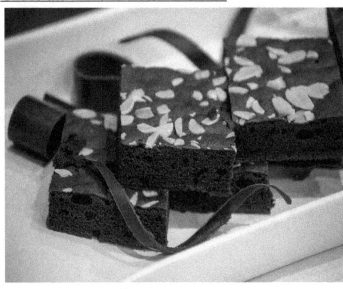

Preparation Time: 10 minutes
Cooking Time: 16 minutes
Servings: 4
Ingredients:
- 1 cup bananas, overripe
- 1/2 cup almond butter, melted
- 1 scoop protein powder
- 2 tbsp unsweetened cocoa powder

Directions:
1. Preheat the air fryer to 325 F. Grease air fryer baking pan and set aside.
2. Blend all ingredients in a blender until smooth.
3. Pour batter into the prepared pan and place in the air fryer basket and cook for 16 minutes.
4. Serve and enjoy.

Peanut Butter Fudge

Preparation Time: 10 minutes
Cooking Time: 10 minutes
Servings: 20
Ingredients:
- 1/4 cup almonds, toasted and chopped
- 12 oz smooth peanut butter
- 15 drops liquid stevia
- 3 tbsp coconut oil
- 4 tbsp coconut cream
- Pinch of salt

Directions:
1. Line baking tray with parchment paper.
2. Melt coconut oil in a pan over low heat. Add peanut butter, coconut cream, stevia, and salt in a saucepan. Stir well. Pour fudge mixture into the prepared baking tray and sprinkle chopped almonds on top.
3. Place the tray in the refrigerator for 1 hour or until set.
4. Slice and serve.

Almond Butter Fudge

Preparation Time: 10 minutes
Cooking Time: 10 minutes
Servings: 18
Ingredients:

- 3/4 cup creamy almond butter
- 1 1/2 cups unsweetened chocolate chips

Directions:

1. Line 8*4-inch pan with parchment paper and set aside.
2. Add chocolate chips and almond butter into the double boiler and cook over medium heat until the chocolate-butter mixture is melted. Stir well. Place mixture into the prepared pan and place in the freezer until set.
3. Slice and serve.

Apple Crumble

Preparation Time: 20 minutes
Cooking Time: 25 minutes
Servings: 6
Ingredients:

FOR THE FILLING

- 5 apples, cored and chopped
- ½ cup unsweetened applesauce
- 3 tablespoons unrefined sugar
- 1 teaspoon ground cinnamon
- Pinch sea salt

FOR THE CRUMBLE

- 2 tablespoons almond butter
- 2 tablespoons maple syrup
- 1½ cups rolled oats
- ½ cup walnuts, chopped
- ½ teaspoon ground cinnamon
- 3 tablespoons unrefined granular sugar

Directions:

1. Preheat the oven to 350°F. Put the apples and applesauce in an 8-inch-square baking dish, and sprinkle with the sugar, cinnamon, and salt. Toss to combine.
2. In a medium bowl, mix together the nut butter and maple syrup until smooth and creamy. Add the oats, walnuts, cinnamon, and sugar and stir to coat, using your hands if necessary. (If you have a small food processor, pulse the oats and walnuts together before adding them to the mix.)
3. Sprinkle the topping over the apples and put the dish in the oven.
4. Bake for 20 to 25 minutes, or until the fruit is soft and the topping is lightly browned. Serve warm!

Cashew-Chocolate Truffles

Preparation Time: 15 minutes
Cooking Time: 0 minutes
Servings: 12
Ingredients:

- 1 cup raw cashews, soaked in water overnight
- ¾ cup pitted dates
- 2 tablespoons coconut oil
- 1 cup unsweetened shredded coconut, divided
- 1 to 2 tablespoons cocoa powder, to taste

Directions:

1. In a food processor, combine the cashews, dates, coconut oil, ½ cup of shredded coconut, and cocoa powder. Pulse until fully incorporated; it will resemble chunky cookie dough. Spread the remaining ½ cup of shredded coconut on a plate. Form the mixture into tablespoon-size balls and roll on the plate to cover with the shredded coconut. Transfer to a parchment paper–lined plate or baking sheet. Repeat to make 12 truffles.
2. Place the truffles in the refrigerator for 1 hour. Transfer them to a plate and serve.

Banana Chocolate Cupcakes

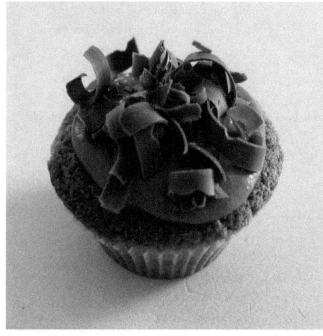

Preparation Time: 20 minutes
Cooking Time: 20 minutes
Servings: 1
Ingredients:

- 3 medium bananas
- 1 cup non-dairy milk
- 2 tablespoons almond butter
- 1 teaspoon apple cider vinegar
- 1 teaspoon pure vanilla extract
- 1¼ cups whole-grain flour
- ½ cup rolled oats
- ¼ cup coconut sugar (optional)
- 1 teaspoon baking powder
- ½ teaspoon baking soda
- ½ cup unsweetened cocoa powder
- ¼ cup chia seeds, or sesame seeds
- Pinch sea salt
- ¼ cup dark chocolate chips, dried cranberries

Directions:

1. Preheat the oven to 350°F. Lightly grease the cups of two 6-cup muffin tins or line with paper muffin cups.
2. Put the bananas, milk, almond butter, vinegar, and vanilla in a blender and purée until smooth. Or stir together in a large bowl until smooth and creamy.
3. Put the flour, oats, sugar (if using), baking powder, baking soda, cocoa powder, chia seeds, salt, and chocolate chips in another large bowl, and stir to combine. Mix together the wet and dry ingredients, stirring as little as possible. Spoon into muffin cups, and bake for 20 to 25 minutes. Take the cupcakes out of the oven and let them cool fully before taking out of the muffin tins, since they'll be very moist.

Minty Fruit Salad

Preparation Time: 3 days 15 minutes
Cooking Time: 5 minutes
Servings: 4
Ingredients:

- ¼ cup lemon juice (about 2 small lemons)
- 4 teaspoons maple syrup or agave syrup
- 2 cups chopped pineapple
- 2 cups chopped strawberries
- 2 cups raspberries
- 1 cup blueberries
- 8 fresh mint leaves

Directions:

1. Beginning with 1 mason jar, add the ingredients in this order: 1 tablespoon of lemon juice, 1 teaspoon of maple syrup, ½ cup of pineapple, ½ cup of strawberries, ½ cup of raspberries, ¼ cup of blueberries, and 2 mint leaves.
2. Repeat to fill 3 more jars. Close the jars tightly with lids.
3. Place the airtight jars in the refrigerator for up to 3 days. Serve!

Mango Coconut Cream Pie

Preparation Time: 20 minutes   **Cooking Time:** 30 minutes   **Servings:** 8
Ingredients: FOR THE CRUST

- ½ cup rolled oats
- 1 cup cashews
- 1 cup soft pitted dates

FOR THE FILLING

- 1 cup canned coconut milk
- ½ cup water
- 2 large mangos, peeled and chopped
- ½ cup unsweetened shredded coconut

Directions:

1. Put all the crust ingredients in a food processor and pulse until it holds together. If you don't have a food processor, chop everything as finely as possible and use ½ cup cashew or almond butter in place of half the cashews. Press the mixture down firmly into an 8-inch pie or springform pan.
2. Put the all filling ingredients in a blender and purée until smooth (about 1 minute). It should be very thick, so you may have to stop and stir until it's smooth.
3. Pour the filling into the crust, use a rubber spatula to smooth the top, and put the pie in the freezer until set, about 30 minutes. Once frozen, it should be set out for about 15 minutes to soften before serving.
4. Top with a batch of Coconut Whipped Cream scooped on top of the pie once it's set. Finish it off with a sprinkling of toasted shredded coconut.

Cherry-Vanilla Rice Pudding (Pressure cooker)

Preparation Time: 5 minutes

Cooking Time: 30 minutes

Servings: 4-6

Ingredients:

- 1 cup short-grain brown rice
- 1¾ cups nondairy milk, plus more as needed
- 1½ cups water
- 4 tablespoons unrefined sugar plus more as needed
- 1 teaspoon vanilla extract
- Pinch salt
- ¼ cup dried cherries

Directions:

1. Preparing the ingredients. In your electric pressure cooker's cooking pot, combine the rice, milk, water, sugar, vanilla, and salt. High pressure for 30 minutes. Close and lock the lid and select High Pressure for 30 minutes.
2. Pressure Release. Once the cooking time is complete, let the pressure release naturally, about 20 minutes. Unlock and remove the lid. Stir in the cherries and put the lid back on loosely for about 10 minutes. Serve, adding more milk or sugar, as desired.

Lime in the Coconut Chia Pudding

Preparation Time: 10 minutes

Cooking Time: 20 minutes

Servings: 4

Ingredients:

- Zest and juice of 1 lime
- 1 (14-ounce) can coconut milk
- 1 to 2 dates
- 2 tablespoons chia seeds, whole or ground
- 2 teaspoons Matcha green tea powder

Directions:

1. Blend all the ingredients in a blender until smooth. Chill in the fridge for about 20 minutes, then serve topped with one or more of the topping ideas.
2. Try blueberries, blackberries, sliced strawberries, Coconut Whipped Cream, or toasted unsweetened coconut.

Mint Chocolate Chip Sorbet

Preparation Time: 5 minutes   **Cooking Time:** 0 minutes   **Servings:** 1

Ingredients:

- 1 frozen banana
- 1 tablespoon almond butter

- 2 tablespoons fresh mint, minced
- ¼ cup or less non-dairy milk
- 2 to 3 tablespoons non-dairy chocolate chips
- 2 to 3 tablespoons goji berries (optional)

Directions:

1. Put the banana, almond butter, and mint in a food processor or blender and purée until smooth.
2. Add the non-dairy milk if needed to keep blending (but only if needed, as this will make the texture less solid). Pulse the chocolate chips and goji berries into the mix so they're roughly chopped up. Serve.

Peach-Mango Crumble (Pressure cooker)

Preparation Time: 10 minutes
Cooking Time: 6 minutes
Servings: 4-6
Ingredient:

- 3 cups chopped peaches
- 3 cups chopped mangos
- 4 tablespoons unrefined sugar divided
- 1 cup gluten-free rolled oats
- ½ cup shredded coconut, unsweetened
- 2 tablespoons coconut oil

Directions:

1. In a 6- to 7-inch round baking dish, toss together the peaches, mangos, and 2 tablespoons of sugar. In a food processor, combine the oats, coconut, coconut oil, and remaining 2 tablespoons of sugar. Pulse until combined. (If you use maple syrup, you'll need less coconut oil. Start with just the syrup and add oil if the mixture isn't sticking together.) Sprinkle the oat mixture over the fruit mixture.
2. Cover the dish with aluminum foil. Put a trivet in the bottom of your electric pressure cooker's cooking pot and pour in a cup or two of water. Using a foil sling or silicone helper handles, lower the pan onto the trivet.
3. High pressure for 6 minutes. Close and lock the lid and select High Pressure for 6 minutes.
4. Once the cooking time is complete, quick release the pressure. Unlock and remove the lid. Let cool for a few minutes before carefully lifting out the dish with oven mitts or tongs. Scoop out portions to serve.

Zesty Orange-Cranberry Energy Bites

Preparation Time: 10 minutes
Cooking Time: 15 minutes
Servings: 12
Ingredients:

- 2 tablespoons almond butter
- 2 tablespoons maple syrup
- ¾ cup cooked quinoa
- ¼ cup sesame seeds, toasted
- 1 tablespoon chia seeds
- ½ teaspoon almond extract
- Zest of 1 orange
- 1 tablespoon dried cranberries
- ¼ cup ground almonds

Directions:

1. In a medium bowl, mix together the nut or seed butter and syrup until smooth and creamy. Stir in the rest of the ingredients and mix to make sure the consistency is holding together in a ball. Form the mix into 12 balls.
2. Place them on a baking sheet lined with parchment or waxed paper and put in the fridge to set for about 15 minutes. If your balls aren't holding together, it's likely because of the moisture content of your cooked quinoa. Add more nut or seed butter mixed with syrup until it all sticks together. Serve.

Almond-Date Energy Bites

Preparation Time: 5 minutes
Cooking Time: 15 minutes
Servings: 24
Ingredients:
Directions:

- 1 cup dates, pitted
- 1 cup shredded coconut
- ¼ cup chia seeds
- ¾ cup ground almonds
- ¼ cup cocoa nibs

1. Purée everything in a food processor until crumbly and sticking together, pushing down the sides whenever necessary to keep it blending. If you don't have a food processor, you can mash soft Medjool dates. But if you're using harder baking dates, you'll have to soak them and then try to purée them in a blender.
2. Form the mix into 24 balls and place them on a baking sheet lined with parchment or waxed paper. Put in the fridge to set for about 15 minutes. Use the softest dates you can find. Medjool dates are the best for this purpose. The hard dates you see in the baking aisle of your supermarket are going to take a long time to blend up. If you use those, try soaking them in water for at least an hour before you start, and then draining.

Pumpkin Pie Cups (Pressure cooker)
Preparation Time: 5 minutes
Cooking Time: 6 minutes
Servings: 4-6
Ingredients:
- 1 cup canned pumpkin purée
- 1 cup nondairy milk
- 6 tablespoons + 1 unrefined sugar
- ¼ cup spelt flour or whole-grain flour
- ½ teaspoon pumpkin pie spice
- Pinch salt

Directions:
1. In a medium bowl, stir together the pumpkin, milk, sugar, flour, pumpkin pie spice, and salt. Pour the mixture into 4 heat-proof ramekins. Sprinkle a bit more sugar on the top of each, if you like. Put a trivet in the bottom of your electric pressure cooker's cooking pot and pour in a cup or two of water. Place the ramekins onto the trivet, stacking them if needed (3 on the bottom, 1 on top). High pressure for 6 minutes. Close and lock the lid and select High Pressure for 6 minutes. Once the cooking time is complete, quick release the pressure. Unlock and remove the lid. Let cool for a few minutes before carefully lifting out the ramekins with oven mitts or tongs. Let cool for at least 10 minutes before serving. Top with sugar and serve.

Coconut and Almond Truffles
Preparation Time: 1 hour 15 minutes
Cooking Time: 0 minutes
Servings: 8
Ingredients:
- 1 cup pitted dates
- 1 cup almonds
- ½ cup sweetened cocoa powder, plus extra
- ½ cup unsweetened shredded coconut
- ¼ cup pure maple syrup
- 1 teaspoon vanilla extract
- 1 teaspoon almond extract
- ¼ teaspoon sea salt

Directions:
1. In the bowl of a food processor, combine all the ingredients and process until smooth. Chill the mixture for about 1 hour. Roll the mixture into balls and then roll the balls in cocoa powder to coat.
2. Serve immediately or keep chilled until ready to serve.

Fudgy Brownies (Pressure cooker)
Preparation Time: 10 minutes
Cooking Time: 5 minutes
Servings: 4-6
Ingredients:
- 3 ounces dark chocolate
- 1 tablespoon coconut oil
- ½ cup applesauce
- 2 tablespoons unrefined sugar
- 1/3 cup whole-grain flour
- ½ teaspoon baking powder
- Pinch salt

Directions:
1. Put a trivet in your electric pressure cooker's cooking pot and pour in a cup or two of two of water. Select Sauté

or Simmer. In a large heat-proof glass or ceramic bowl, combine the chocolate and coconut oil. Place the bowl over the top of your pressure cooker, as you would a double boiler.

2. Stir occasionally until the chocolate is melted, then turn off the pressure cooker. Stir the applesauce and sugar into the chocolate mixture. Add the flour, baking powder, and salt and stir just until combined. Pour the batter into 3 heat-proof ramekins. Put them in a heat-proof dish and cover with aluminum foil. Using a foil sling or silicone helper handles, lower the dish onto the trivet. (Alternately, cover each ramekin with foil and place them directly on the trivet, without the dish.)

3. High pressure for 6 minutes. Close and lock the lid and select High Pressure for 5 minutes.

4. Pressure Release. Once the cooking time is complete, quick release the pressure. Unlock and remove the lid.

5. Let cool for a few minutes before carefully lifting out the dish, or ramekins, with oven mitts or tongs. Let cool for a few minutes more before serving. Top with fresh raspberries and an extra drizzle of melted chocolate.

Chocolate Macaroons

Preparation Time: 10 minutes
Cooking Time: 15 minutes
Servings: 8
Ingredients:

- 1 cup unsweetened shredded coconut
- 2 tablespoons cocoa powder
- 2/3 cup coconut milk
- ¼ cup agave
- pinch of sea salt

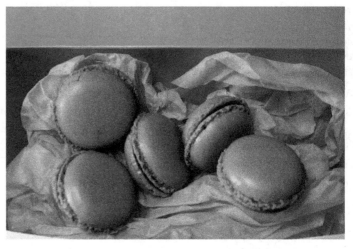

Directions:

1. Preheat the oven to 350°F. Line a baking sheet with parchment paper. In a medium saucepan, cook all the ingredients over -medium-high heat until a firm dough is formed. Scoop the dough into balls and place on the baking sheet. Bake for 15 minutes, remove from the oven, and let cool on the baking sheet.

2. Serve cooled macaroons or store in a tightly sealed container.

Mandarin Cream

Preparation Time: 30 minutes
Cooking Time: 0 minutes
Servings: 8
Ingredients:

- 2 mandarins, peeled and cutted

- Juice of 2 mandarins
- 2 tablespoons stevia
- 4 eggs, whisked
- ¾ cup stevia
- ¾ cup almonds, ground

Directions:

1. In a blender, combine the mandarins with the mandarin's juice and the other ingredients, whisk well, divide into cups.

2. Keep in the fridge for 20 minutes before serving.

Creamy Mint Strawberry Mix

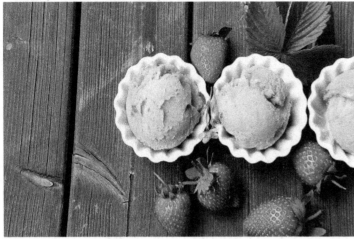

Preparation Time: 10 minutes
Cooking Time: 30 minutes
Servings: 6
Ingredients:
- Cooking spray
- ¼ cup stevia
- 1 and ½ cup almond flour
- 1 teaspoon baking powder
- 1 cup almond milk
- 1 egg, whisked
- 2 cups strawberries, sliced
- 1 tablespoon mint, chopped
- 1 teaspoon lime zest, grated
- ½ cup whipping cream

Directions:
1. In a bowl, combine the almond with the strawberries, mint and the other ingredients except the cooking spray and whisk well.
2. Grease 6 ramekins with the cooking spray, pour the strawberry mix inside, place in the oven and bake at 350°F for 30 minutes. Cool down and serve.

Vanilla Cake

Preparation Time: 10 minutes
Cooking Time: 25 minutes
Servings: 10
Ingredients:
- 3 cups almond flour
- 3 teaspoons baking powder
- 1 cup olive oil
- 1 and ½ cup almond milk
- 1 and 2/3 cup stevia
- 2 cups water
- 1 tablespoon lime juice
- 2 teaspoons vanilla extract
- Cooking spray

Directions:
1. In a bowl, mix the almond flour with the baking powder, the oil and the rest of the ingredients except the cooking spray and whisk well.
2. Pour the mix into a cake pan greased with the cooking spray, introduce in the oven and bake at 370 degrees F for 25 minutes. Leave the cake to cool down, cut and serve!

Pumpkin Cream

Preparation Time: 5 minutes
Cooking Time: 5 minutes
Servings: 2
Ingredients:
- 2 cups canned pumpkin flesh
- 2 tablespoons stevia
- 1 teaspoon vanilla extract
- 2 tablespoons water
- A pinch of pumpkin spice

Directions:
1. In a pan, combine the pumpkin flesh with the other ingredients, simmer for 5 minutes.
2. Divide into cups and serve cold.

Chia and Berries Smoothie Bowl

Preparation Time: 5 minutes
Cooking Time: 0 minutes
Servings: 2
Ingredients:

- 1 and ½ cup almond milk
- 1 cup blackberries
- ¼ cup strawberries, chopped
- 1 and ½ tablespoons chia seeds
- 1 teaspoon cinnamon powder

Directions:

1. In a blender, combine the blackberries with the strawberries and the rest of the ingredients, pulse well, divide into small bowls and serve cold.

Minty Coconut Cream

Preparation Time: 4 minutes
Cooking Time: 0 minutes
Servings: 2
Ingredients:

- 1 banana, peeled
- 2 cups coconut flesh, shredded
- 3 tablespoons mint, chopped
- 1 and ½ cups coconut water
- 2 tablespoons stevia
- ½ avocado, pitted and peeled

Directions:

1. In a blender, combine the coconut with the banana and the rest of the ingredients, pulse well.
2. Divide into cups and serve cold.

Grapes Stew

Preparation Time: 10 minutes
Cooking Time: 10 minutes
Servings: 4
Ingredients:

- 2/3 cup stevia
- 1 tablespoon olive oil
- 1/3 cup coconut water
- 1 teaspoon vanilla extract
- 1 teaspoon lemon zest, grated
- 2 cup red grapes, halved

Directions:

1. Heat up a pan with the water over medium heat, add the oil, stevia and the rest of the ingredients, toss, simmer for 10 minutes, divide into cups and serve.

Nutrient Protein Salad Recipes

Quinoa and Chickpea Salad

Preparation Time: 10 Minutes

Cooking Time: 0 Minutes

Servings: 4

Ingredients:

- 2 cups cooked quinoa
- 1½ cups canned red beans, drained
- 3 cups fresh baby spinach
- ¼ cup sun-dried tomatoes, chopped
- ¼ cup fresh dill
- ¼ cup fresh parsley
- ½ cup sunflower seeds
- ¼ cup walnuts, chopped
- 3 tablespoons fresh lemon juice
- Salt and black pepper to taste

Directions:

1. In a large bowl, add all the ingredients and toss to coat well.
2. Serve immediately.

Mixed Grain Salad

Preparation Time: 20 Minutes

Cooking Time: 0 Minutes

Servings: 6

Ingredients:

DRESSING

- ¼ cup fresh lime juice
- 2 tablespoons maple syrup
- 1 tablespoon Dijon mustard
- ½ teaspoon ground cumin
- 1 teaspoon garlic powder
- Salt and black pepper, to taste
- ½ cup extra-virgin olive oil

SALAD

- 2 cups fresh mango, peeled, and cubed
- 2 tablespoon fresh lime juice, divided
- 2 avocados, peeled, pitted, and cubed
- Pinch of salt
- 1 cup cooked quinoa
- 2 cans black beans, drained
- 1 can corn, drained
- 1 small red onion, chopped
- 1 jalapeño, seeded and chopped
- ½ cup fresh cilantro, chopped
- 6 cups romaine lettuce, shredded

Directions:

1. For dressing: in a blender, add all the ingredients (except oil) and pulse until well combined. While the motor is running, gradually add the oil and pulse until smooth.
2. For salad: in a bowl, add the mango and 1 tablespoon of lime juice and toss to coat well. In another bowl, add the avocado, a pinch of salt, and remaining lime juice and toss to coat well.
3. In a large serving bowl, add the mango, avocado, and remaining salad ingredients and mix.
4. Place the dressing and toss to coat well. Serve immediately.

Rice and Tofu Salad

Preparation Time: 15 Minutes   **Cooking Time:** 0 Minutes   **Servings:** 4   **Ingredients:**

SALAD:

- 12-ounce tofu, pressed, drained, and sliced
- 1½ cups cooked brown rice
- 3 large tomatoes, peeled and chopped
- ¼ cup fresh basil leaves

DRESSING:

- 3 scallions, chopped
- 2 tablespoons black sesame seeds, toasted
- 2 tablespoons low-sodium soy sauce
- ½ teaspoon sesame oil, toasted
- Drop of hot pepper sauce
- 1 tablespoon maple syrup
- ¼ teaspoon red chili powder

Directions:
1. In a large serving bowl, place all the ingredients and toss to coat well. Serve immediately.

Kidney Bean and Pomegranate Salad

Preparation Time: 15 Minutes
Cooking Time: 0 Minutes
Servings: 3
Ingredients:

- 2 cups canned white kidney beans, drained
- 1 cup fresh pomegranate seeds
- 1/3 cup scallion chopped
- 2 tablespoons fresh parsley, chopped
- 1 tablespoon fresh lime juice
- Salt and pepper to taste

Directions:
1. In a large serving bowl, place all the ingredients and toss to coat well. Serve immediately.

Warm Vegetable Salad

Preparation Time: 25 Minutes
Cooking Time: 0 Minutes
Servings: 4
Ingredients:

- Cashew cream (1 c.)
- Pepper
- Dried dill (2 teaspoons)
- Lime juice (2 Tablespoons)
- Olive oil (1 Tablespoon)
- Sliced carrots (1 lb.)
- Quartered red potatoes
- Salt

Directions:
1. Bring some salted water to a pot and add in the potatoes. After 8 minutes of cooking, add in the carrots and cook until these are done. Drain out the water. In the pot before, without the water, add in the oil, dill, salt, and lime juice and stir to combine. Divide these between four containers and then top with the cream before serving.

Not-Tuna Salad

Preparation Time: 5 Minutes
Cooking Time: 0 Minutes
Servings: 4
Ingredients:

- Pepper (25 teaspoons)
- Salt (5 teaspoons)
- Vegan mayo (25 c.)
- Diced celery (5 c.)
- Chopped white onion (5 c.)
- Hearts of palm (1 can)
- Chickpeas (1 can)

Directions:
1. Bring out a bowl and use a potato masher to help mash up the chickpeas to make chunky. Add in the pepper, salt, vegan mayo, celery, onion, and hearts of palm. Combine and add in some more mayo if you would like.
2. Divide into four servings and serve or save for later.

Corn and Red Bean Salad

Preparation Time: 15 Minutes   **Cooking Time:** 0 Minutes   **Servings:** 4
Ingredients:

- Chopped Romaine lettuce (8 c)

- Barley (1 c.)
- Corn (2 c.)
- Kidney beans (2 cans)
- Chili powder (1 teaspoon.)
- Cashew cream (25 c.)

Directions:
1. Take out some quart jars and set them out. In a small bowl, whisk the chili powder and cream.
2. Pour a bit of this cream into each jar and then add in some of the kidney beans, corn, and cooked barley.
3. Add in two cups of the romaine and then punch down to fit into the jar well. close the lids and then enjoy.

Tabbouleh Salad

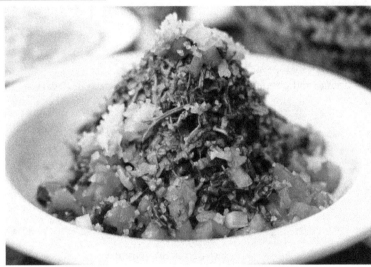

Preparation Time: 25 Minutes
Cooking Time: 0 Minutes
Servings: 4
Ingredients:
- Sunflower seeds (4 Tablespoons)
- Chopped scallions
- Chopped mint (25 c.)
- Chopped parsley (1 c.)
- Diced tomato
- Diced cucumber
- Olive oil (1 Tablespoon)
- Salt
- Pressed garlic cloves
- Zest and juice of one lemon
- Boiling water (1 c.)
- Couscous (1 c.)

Directions:
1. Put the couscous into a bowl and cover with the boiling water. Cover and set aside. Add the lemon juice and zest to a bowl and stir in the olive oil, salt, and garlic. Put the scallions, mint, parsley, tomato, and cucumber into the bowl and toss to coat with the dressing.
2. Take the plate off the couscous and fluff with the fork. Add this to the vegetables and toss to combine.

Cauliflower and Apple Salad

Preparation Time: 25 minutes
Cooking Time: 0 minutes
Servings: 4
Ingredients:
- 3 cups cauliflower chopped
- 2 cups Baby Kale
- 1 apple cored and chopped
- ¼ cup basil chopped
- ¼ cup mint chopped
- ¼ cup parsley chopped
- ¼ cup scallions sliced
- 2 tablespoons yellow raisins
- 1 tablespoon sun dried tomatoes chopped
- ¼ cup roasted pumpkin seeds, optional

Directions:
1. Take a bowl and mix all the ingredients.
2. Sprinkle pumpkin seeds on top and serve. Enjoy!

Corn and Black Bean Salad

Preparation Time: 25 minutes   **Cooking Time:** 0 minutes   **Servings:** 6
Ingredients:
- ¼ cup cilantro, chopped
- 1 can corn, drained

- ½ red onion, chopped
- 1 can black beans, drained
- 1 tomato, chopped

- 3 tablespoons lemon juice
- 2 tablespoons olive oil
- Salt and pepper to taste

Directions:

1. Mix everything together in a bowl. Refrigerate for 20 minutes. Serve cold.

Spinach and Orange Salad

Preparation Time: 15 minutes

Cooking Time: 0 minutes

Servings: 6

Ingredients:

- ¼ cup mustard

- 3 oranges peeled
- ¾ lb. spinach, torn
- 1 medium red onion

Directions:

1. Take a bowl and add in sliced onion, chopped orange and chopped spinaches. Mix and add mustard. Serve!

Red Pepper and Broccoli Salad

Preparation Time: 15 minutes

Cooking Time: 0 minutes

Servings: 2

Ingredients:

- 2 cups lettuce salad
- 1 head Broccoli, chopped
- 1 red pepper, seeded

DRESSING:

- 3 tablespoons white wine vinegar
- 1 teaspoon mustard
- 1 garlic clove, peeled
- Salt and pepper to taste
- 2 tablespoons olive oil
- 1 tablespoon parsley, minced

Directions:

1. Take a pot and bring the water to a boil. Season with salt and cook broccoli to 10 minutes. Drain them.
2. Take a bowl, add broccoli, chopped lettuce and chopped pepper. Add wine vinegar, mustard, garlic sliced, olive oil, parsley, a pinch of salt and pepper. Mix well and serve!

Lentil Potato Salad

Preparation Time: 35 minutes

Cooking Time: 25 minutes

Servings: 2

Ingredients:

- ½ cup beluga lentils

- 8 fingerling potatoes
- 1 cup scallions, sliced thin
- ¼ cup cherry tomatoes
- ¼ cup lemon vinaigrette
- salt and pepper to taste

Directions:

1. Bring two cups of water to simmer in a pot and add your lentils.
2. Cook for 20 minutes, and then drain only the lentils. Your lentils should be tender.
3. Reduce to a simmer and add potatoes into the water before. Cook them for 15 minutes, and then drain. Halve your potatoes once they're cool enough to touch.
4. Put your lentils on a serving plate. Top with scallions, chopped potatoes and chopped tomatoes. Drizzle with your vinaigrette, and season with salt and pepper. Enjoy!

21 - Day Meal Plan

Day	Breakfast	Lunch	Dinner	Snacks/Desserts
1	Lean & Green Smoothie	Curry Soup	Herbed Beets	Orange Ricotta Pancake
2	Mango Cucumber Smoothie	Green Pea Fritter	Zucchini Soup	Chocolate Bars
3	Cream Cheese Egg Breakfast	Tuna Cakes	Mustard Beets	Chia Pudding
4	Broccoli Orange Smoothie	Polenta Seared Pears	Mixed Grain salad	Vitamin C Smoothie Cubes
5	Avocado and Cucumber Smoothie	Buttery Broccoli and Bacon	Moroccan Vermicelli Vegetable Soup	Chocolate Almond Butter Brownie
6	Avocado Red Pepper Roasted Scrambled Egg	Tomato Braised Cauliflower Chicken	Avocado Cucumber Soup	Cucumber, Celery Apple Smoothie
7	Kiwi and Mint Smoothie	Taco Stuffed Avocado	Delicious Pizza	Avocado Pudding
8	Apple, Banana, Collard Greens Smoothie	Bacon Spaghetti Squash Carbonara	Turkey Lettuce Wraps	Carrot, Avocado and Tomato Smoothie
	Zucchini Bread Smoothie	Mexican Pork Stew	Cauliflower Crust Pizza	Spicy Pumpkin Muffins
10	Lime Bacon Thyme Muffins	Creamy Curry Noodles	Spinach and Pear Salad	Raspberry Ice Cream
11	Gluten -Free Pancakes	Roasted Vegetables	Olives and Mango Mix	Chocolate Frosty
12		Creamy Squash Soup	Mini Mac in a Bowl	Peach Mango Crumble
13	Tasty Breakfast Donuts	Cauliflower Apple Salad	Spinach and Orange Salad	Black and blueberries smoothie
14	Lean & Green Smoothie 2	Lentil Potato Salad	Marinara Broccoli	Pumpkin Balls
15	Asian Scrambled Egg	Vegetarian Nachos	Cashew Zucchinis	Apple Crumble
16	Artichoke Frittatas	Potato Carrot Salad	Spinach Pear Salad	Peanut Butter cream
17	Chocolate Sweet Potato Pudding	Cilantro Lime Coleslaw	Garlic Beans	Banana Chocolate Cupcakes
18	Pineapple Celery Smoothie	Delicious Broccoli	Mustard Beets	Minty Fruit Salad
19	Zucchini Frittata	Spicy Peanut Noodles	Parsley Green Beans	Mango Coconut Cream Pie
20	Tropical Green Smoothies	Tabbouleh Salad	Avocado Mint Soup	Coconut Coffee and Ghee
21	Mocha Oatmeal	Taco Stuffed Avocados	Bok Choy Salad	Lime in the Coconut Chia Pudding

This is an example of a 21-day Meal Plan. You can change these foods.

Conclusion

Thank you for reading this book!

I hope these recipes can help you start healthy habits by eating delicious meals!

As I said at the beginning of this book, I created this book to allow busy people to eat healthy *without sacrificing taste*!

Regardless of what diet people may be on, the key is to vary foods and get the right amount of daily nutrients!

The key to maintaining weight and preventing disease is ***having healthy habits*** - this includes a *healthy lifestyle*, a *balanced diet*, and *regular exercise*.

I suggest you follow this easy 21-meal plan to start creating your healthy habits and get about 30 minutes of gentle exercise each day. ***It's a great way to start your journey to health!***

Thanks very much for reading, and I wish you to achieve all your goals!

Michelle Laurie Johnson

CPSIA information can be obtained
at www.ICGtesting.com
Printed in the USA
BVHW060730010521
606210BV00007B/1797